Primitive Surgery

An Overview

Ana Doria Buchan

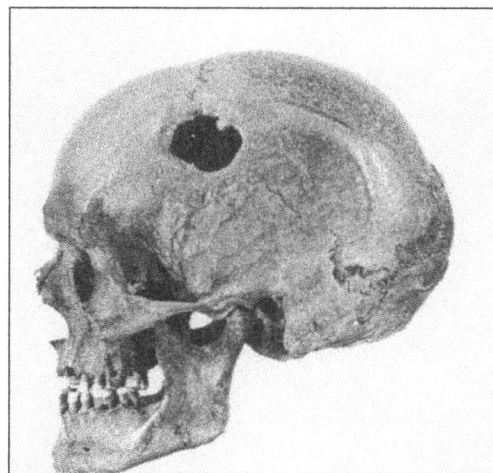

BAR International Series 1512
2006

Published in 2019 by
BAR Publishing, Oxford

BAR International Series 1512

Primitive Surgery

© A D Buchan and the Publisher 2006

ISBN 9781841717470 paperback
ISBN 9781407329666 e-book

DOI https://doi.org/10.30861/9781841717470

A catalogue record for this book is available from the British Library

This book is available at www.barpublishing.com

BAR Publishing is the trading name of British Archaeological Reports (Oxford) Ltd.
British Archaeological Reports was first incorporated in 1974 to publish the BAR
Series, International and British. In 1992 Hadrian Books Ltd became part of the BAR
group. This volume was originally published by John and Erica Hedges Ltd. in
conjunction with British Archaeological Reports (Oxford) Ltd / Hadrian Books Ltd,
the Series principal publisher, in 2006. This present volume is published by BAR
Publishing, 2019.

BAR
PUBLISHING

BAR titles are available from:

BAR Publishing
122 Banbury Rd, Oxford, OX2 7BP, UK
EMAIL   info@barpublishing.com
PHONE   +44 (0)1865 310431
FAX   +44 (0)1865 316916
www.barpublishing.com

Primitive Surgery

TABLE OF CONTENTS

I – ACKNOWLEDGEMENTS

I would like to thank Dr Tony Waldron for making my passion for archaeology expand to the surgery field and Wendy Birch for her kind and professional help. I also wish to show much gratitude to my parents and husband, for their patience and love.

II – ABSTRACT

Surgery, from the Greek kheirourgia - "handiwork", is the branch of medicine concerned with treatment of disease, injury or deformity of the body by manual or instrumental operative procedures, and is as old as mankind. Having played a central role in health and healing throughout the ages, the ideas and methods of surgery are fascinating from many points of view.

As the following will show, although the surgery of primitive peoples has held, even in the most ancient periods, an astonishing degree of technical efficiency, it has remained fairly undeveloped and limited in scope. This is due to the fact that although technical in character, this science is determined by the concept of disease prevailing in a given society. Since it aims at removing the disease by cutting out the diseased part or at restoring disturbed anatomical conditions, it seems apparent that surgery could not fully develop before the 19th century, when medicine finally accepted an anatomical concept of disease. The pain, pus, blood and disfigurement associated with surgery undermined the acceptance of this form of treatment for millennia, and as long as medicine looked upon illness as a disturbance in the equilibrium of the body's humours (liquids), surgery could not be more than a last resort for physicians when all other treatments had failed.

The two events that mark the beginning of modern surgery are the introduction of anaesthesia and of the antiseptic system, which means that modern surgery is really not much more than a century old.

Accordingly, present-day knowledge and techniques have resulted from the cumulative observations and experiments of millennia.

1. __INTRODUCTION__

Disease has always been an inseparable companion of life. Man has been subject to disease from the time of his first appearance on the stage of prehistory some 500,000 years ago. The human body has been constantly exposed to assault and injury, invasion by parasites, extremes of heat and cold, and infections. It is also probable that early man suffered from a various number of diseases due to nutritional factors and disorders of the body chemistry such as cancer, sinusitis, tumours, tuberculosis, congenital dislocations, and fractures.

Consequently, surgery in some form has developed to a greater or lesser extent in all cultures. Although there is no way of knowing when the earliest surgical operations were performed, it is reasonable to assume that frequent attempts were accomplished by our most distant prehistoric ancestors. Thus, there is no reason to doubt that possibly 250 thousand years ago *Homo sapiens* was already carrying out such manipulations in order to assuage injuries and diseases. Prehistoric man was indeed a skilful craftsman, and we should not be surprised if he had applied his skill to surgical operations.

Pain releases a series of instinctive actions, some of which are more effective than others. This innate instinct for self-preservation is present among all mammals and can lead a dog to lick its wounds or a cat to seek out purging. We can imagine early man suffering an acute pain in the stomach and feeling impelled to act, pressing his epigastrium with both hands, applying heat or cold, drinking water or some decoction until he felt relieved. Eventually, he would learn to differentiate between treatments and pass them on, and a body of empirical medical lore would be acquired, becoming the common knowledge of the group.

Thus, beginning as a response to simple injury, the earliest techniques of surgery were presumably the splinting of fractures, the control of bleeding by pressure, and the removal of foreign bodies such as thorns and splinters. From there it was a reasonable step to open and drain a swollen abscess and, by analogy, to relieve a headache by bleeding.

Procedures such as tattooing, production of tribal marks and scars, piercing of the nose or ears, splitting of the lips and similar ritual operations cannot be considered as surgery in the strict sense of the word, *i.e.*, treatment of disease, injury or deformity of the body, and will therefore not be mentioned in this book.

Regrettably, evidence of diseases or injuries to soft tissue during prehistory has rotted away with the debris of time, which means that skeletal remains provide the most informative sources of evidence for surgery. Written and artistic sources can provide supporting information, but should be used with great caution, given that they might be subject to the bias of an author or artist who may select which aspects of the operation to describe or depict. Such representations are also determined by cultural factors such as ideology. For this reason, I decided not to mention any written sources such as the Egyptian Medical Papyri, the Code of Hammurabi, or the Talmud; I will stick to prehistoric skeletal material and contemporary ethnical reports.

To this extent, we do not have a great amount of information on how these surgical operations were conducted by prehistoric man. The practises of numerous present-day non-industrialised societies nevertheless provide indirect information about surgical achievements accomplished by early humans. We can therefore try and make guesses at what prehistoric healers used to do from studies carried out by anthropologists who, mainly around the end of the nineteenth – beginnings of the twentieth century studied the lives of certain communities all over the world who had never had contact with the so-called "modern man". Archaeology and Anthropology, although using different methods and materials, deal with the same fundamental features of human behaviour; therefore data taken from modern primitives often provide valuable checks or confirmations for general conclusions reached on the basis of archaeological material. On the other hand, anthropologists can benefit greatly from consulting archaeological data. The treatments conducted by such widespread communities certainly match to some degree the care given by our most primitive ancestors. I would like to point out at this stage that by "modern primitives" I mean hunter-gatherer non-industrialised societies; there is no judgement attached to the former expression, it is just a diminutive for the latter.

Nonetheless, the problem is not quite so simple: on one hand, modern primitive societies are very different from one another; on the other, they are not static, and we also know that the development of culture in various parts of the world did not always pass through the same stages, from stone to bronze and iron, from basketry to pottery, and so on. Modern primitive communities stand apart from the main current of evolution of medicine initiated by the Greeks based on rigorous logic, experimentation and recorded observation. Moreover, there are very few primal cultures today which have not reacted to the impact of modern civilisation. It is impossible, therefore, to accept the evolutionary theory of culture integrally and to identify without further ado medicine of today's primitives with prehistoric medicine.

However, the effectiveness of medicine can be measured and expressed in figures, and hence we can certainly distinguish between primitive and advanced conditions. There is no doubt that the beginnings of medicine were primitive everywhere and that conditions were probably similar in many ways to those we find among some of today's primitive peoples; though contemporary tribal men cannot be equated with prehistoric man, they resemble them more than modernised men do.

The purpose of this book is then to analyse the present state of knowledge on when primitive man began to practise surgery, as well as the main characteristics of this branch of medicine in modern primitive societies, a whole vast subject which unfortunately is largely a matter of conjecture.

2. WOUND TREATMENT

A wound is an injury to living tissue by a cut or blow resulting in the piercing of the skin. On account of their lifestyle, prehistoric man quickly became familiar with the sight of wounds; prehistoric man even left pictures of himself pierced by arrows, and all cultures, in some way or other, treat them. As Ackerknecht (1967) points out, such action is in general regarded as "good" by modern primitives.

Majno (1975) describes the remains of an *Australopithecus africanus* whose three and a half million year-old skull probably bears witness to the "first wound". The bones show peculiar depressions that have been interpreted as evidence of an attack with a weapon.

There are various technical procedures in the course of wound treatment: the dressing, the suturing, the drainage, and the stemming of blood flow.

Surgical dressing must have had its common origin in necessity. The first thing a wounded man would do certainly was to protect it from the influence of external forces or agents by the application and maintenance on the surface of the wound of various substances. The first dressing ever used may have been the leaf of a tree or shrub. Some substances were found to be less painful when applied than others; some gave better protection and results. Many things were tried and many observations were made; in time a corpus of experience accumulated and was passed on orally to others for use in similar situations - a considerable sum of empirical knowledge was gradually acquired. Primitive wound dressings often contained components which might have functioned as astringents and antiseptics; others contained pharmacologically valuable ingredients. Yet, symbolic values were likely to predominate. Some North American Indians often applied hot leaves or packed the wound with hot sand, eagle down or scrapings from the inside of tanned hides, while the Dakota tribes seem to have washed them out with a kind of syringe made of a bladder and the quill of a feather, then draining by inserting wicks of soft tree bark into their wounds. The Melanesians applied a bandage of tapa cloth tightly to the bleeding part (Magner, 1992). The Aleut Eskimos dress their wounds with pieces of gut to keep the sea water from wetting them and then dust the wounds with powdered teeth and cover them with the fresh skin of a mouse (Fortuine, 1985). While tar formed an old favourite folk dressing in Europe, most Australian tribes employ clay as a surgical dressing, while the Aborigines of East Arnhem use the stalk of the *cicad*, which is cut into small pieces, placed in a paper-bark basket, mixed with urine, warmed by dropping a hot stone into it, and then applied to the wound. The natives of Victoria in Australia looked upon bleeding with favour as it cleansed the wound. They encouraged the flow by suction, changes in posture, and kneading the tissues, then laid upon it a lump of resin as a dressing (Webb, 1933). Among the Mano of Liberia deep flesh wounds were treated by washing them with leaves of *combretum sp.* boiled in water; the wound is then closed and the remainder of the leaves used as a poultice (Harley, 1970).

The suturing of a wound is the joining of its edges by stitching. Since animal skins were in prehistoric times sewn together for clothing, it is likely that human skin lacerations were sutured as well. Bone needles furnished with an eye, together with the tools used in their manufacture, have been found in French and English Palaeolithic deposits. They had been made by taking a splinter from a bone and then rounding it by scraping with a serrated flint (Bishop, 1960). North American Indians used threads of deer sinews on bone needles for such purpose. The needles were left in and the thread twisted around them (a kind of skewer method which was used in the western world in operations for the cure of harelip as late as the eighteenth century). The same kind of method is encountered in Uganda, while the Kenyan Akamba used thorns (Ackerknecht, 1967). The only tribe known to suture vessels is the Masai of Southeast Africa, who do it with tendons. Long white acacia thorns are passed through the skin and muscular tissue well back from the border of the wound and out through the opposite side. A path for the thorn is made by means of a sharp awl, and a strip of tough vegetable fibre is then wound around the protruding edges of the thorn in a figure of eight, the surfaces of the wound being thus brought fairly well together. The edges of the skin are then more carefully

5

pierced with the awl and brought neatly together by a series of close stitches tied with a reef knot. It has been reported that sword slashes and spear stabs sewn up in this way often do well (Bishop, 1960; Harley, 1970). I take the opportunity to point out that the surgery of this African tribe is in fact much more superior to that of all other primitive tribes reported. An ingenious method devised by surgeons in East Africa, India, and Brazil requires particular species of termites or ants: the insects are brought in contact with the wound and stimulated to bite through its edges, whereupon their heads are cut off and the jaws remain as "suture clamps" (Rogers, 1985; Magner, 1992). The powerful jaws of the insect thus act like the pincers or clips used in modern surgery. Suturing is widely practised in Alaska; when a member of the Aleut tribe injures his body, he grasps the injured place with his hand while another man sews up the wound with a bone needle and thread made of animal veins; on Nunivak Island deep cuts are sutured with human hair (Fortuine, 1985).

The drainage of wounds is the process of drawing off liquid or removing purulent matter, a procedure which is mainly reported from North American Indians. The need to create an outlet where pus has collected is an old rule and there is no reason to doubt that our prehistoric ancestors did not realise its value. How this can be done with primitive means is shown by the Dakota Indians, who sharpen a feather-quill and mount it on an animal's bladder; the quill is then stuck into the afflicted area and the pus is sucked up into the bladder (Haeger, 1988). The same principle is still followed today, the difference being that we use rubber tubes. These tribes are indeed known to be extremely cautious with keeping the wounds clean, and in their clashes with the white men their wound treatment often gave better results than that of their enemies. One of the most remarkable aspects of their medicine is the use of some form of aseptic technique; the Illinois Indians pour into a wound some warm water with diluted drugs, and the results are reported to be quite efficient (Wyatt, 1994). The Aleuts treat wounds by a complete fast lasting from two to four days, since they believe that a minimum of food or drink would cause the wound to become inflamed; in older wounds, warm fish oil or fat from the skull bones of the fox are used for cleansing. The Nunamiut Eskimos put seal oil and spruce gum locally on a wound to prevent infection (Fortuine, 1985), while the Australians of Victoria opt for the method of sucking the wound (Sigerist, 1951).

Haemostasis, or stopping the blood flow, must have been a difficult problem for primitives, who would have used such diverse materials as powdered gum, charcoal, ashes, eagle down, and bandages of bark or coconut fibre. The Algerian Berbers of Aures Massif apply ashes of paper, powdered leaves, pieces of dirty wool dipped in olive oil (it is interesting to draw attention to the fact that dirty wool was used by European surgeons as late as the 19th century), dried goats dung, damp earth and powdered gallnut for such purpose (Ackerknecht, 1967; Bishop, 1960). Among the Mano, if there is severe haemorrhage, dry dust from the ground is sprinkled on the wound to stop the bleeding, and sometimes fresh cow dung is also used. The reason for this is not understood, but according to Harley (1970), it is possible that the type of organisms thus introduced are less virulent than some which might be introduced by ordinary dirt. The Aleut Eskimos control bleeding by immersing the cut in urine or applying tobacco leaves to a fresh wound, while the Koniags apply a powder made from rotten fir wood (Fortuine, 1985). Excess bleeding is arrested by North American Indians by spider webs or pulverised puffballs (Vogel, 1970). Various tribes in Africa, North America and Oceania are familiar with the use of tourniquets, a device for stopping the flow of blood through an artery by twisting a bar in a ligature or bandage (Ackerknecht, 1967).

One of the most common styptic methods, widely practised in present-day Africa and Oceania, is nevertheless cauterisation, which is the burning of tissue with a heated instrument or caustic substance. Used primarily to control haemorrhage, it serves also as an antiputrefactive agent, minimising suppuration, and was probably the first application of the principle of debridement, *i.e.*, the removal of damaged tissue or foreign matter from a wound. In many African tribes, cautery with a hot iron is used to blister a painful spot or to open abscesses. Neck tumours were cauterised in Zimbabwe while in Uganda the operation was executed as a cure for pneumonia. In treating ragged wounds, the Banyankole of Central Africa heat a spear point and work it inside the wound to stop the bleeding and to burn out any unhealthy tissue. Cauterisation might have had a folkloristic origin in the sense that the worship of fire was quite general among primitive peoples and the application of the iron that had just been heated could have been thought to bring such power to aid in curing the ailment. According to Rogers (1985), cauterization was surely given more connotation than its role as a haemostatic agent could justify.

3. FRACTURES

A fracture is the result of any traumatic incident that leads to a partial or complete break of a bone. It surely faced all societies in the past and it would have presented many problems, since it is not only painful but also debilitating. Evidence for the treatment of trauma is plentiful in both anthropological and archaeological data. As in the case of wounds, numerous reports on primitive people emphasise the good treatment of fractures.

Fractures are classified as closed or open (compound) and simple or multi-fragmentary (comminuted). Closed fractures are those in which the skin is intact, while compound fractures involve wounds that communicate with the fracture and may expose bone to contamination.

The major causes of fracture are acute injury (either accidental or intentional), underlying disease (which weakens the bone leaving it more susceptible to fracture), and repeated stress. This treatment comprises two phases: reduction of the fracture, *i.e.*, to put the ends of the bone back in alignment; and immobilisation, which is done by a variety of techniques, splinting being the most common one.

Satisfactory healing of fractures in adults is a long process, during which time total rest of the injured part is essential. In the past, this may not have been too difficult to do in the case of an upper limb fracture, when the afflicted individual would have been able to perform some tasks with the opposite limb, but it would have been much more difficult in the case of a fractured lower limb bone, particularly in hunter-gatherer populations. "In such cases the injured (…) would have been dependent for welfare upon kinspeople. And what reorganisation of lifestyle of the group would be required if the injured was a member of a nomadic group, for surely he or she would be totally incapacitated for perhaps three months with a badly fractured femur?" (Roberts and

9

Manchester, 1997: 94-95). The injured victim of prehistory must have suffered not only the intense pain of the fractured leg, but also the long period of total immobility and dependence upon others and the subsequent crippling due to a grossly shortened leg.

Bone fractures healing in a position of poor alignment and consequent shortening of the affected limb are in fact a common finding in prehistoric skeletal remains, especially in the case of large bones such as the femur and with comminuted fractures. Webb (1995) reports that among Australian aboriginal skeletal remains, malunification of the femur is much more common than united fractures, while healed tibias show a wide range of variation, with both good and bad examples of shaft alignment.

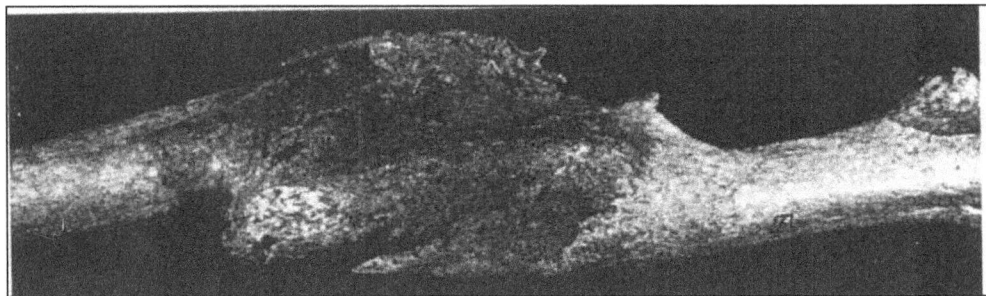

Figure 1 - Fracture of a femoral shaft from Queensland (Australia), which has resulted in a large overlap of the broken ends, shortening the leg considerably

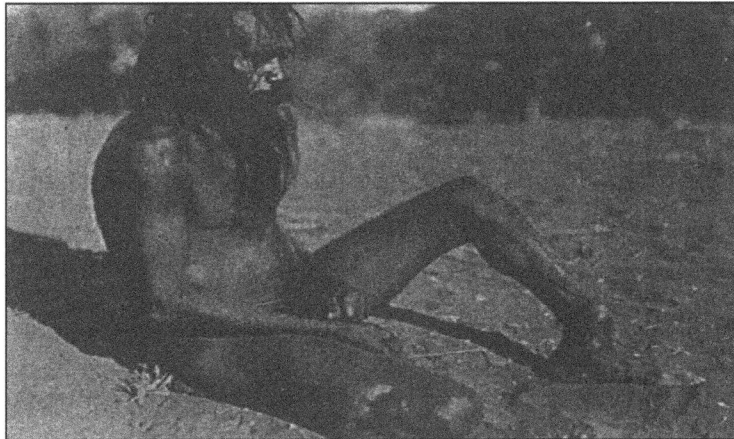

Figure 2 – Man from the Northern Territory (Australia) with a fracture of the lower leg. The deformity must have been overcome to enable him to continue leading a traditional lifestyle

Splints are strips of any rigid material used for holding a broken bone when set, and their use is reported from different cultures all over the world. Notwithstanding, Ackerknecht (1967) stresses that its use does not always prevent bad healing, possibly due to the absence of proper setting of the fragments, *i.e.*, the initial reduction of the fracture not being accurate enough. In my opinion, lack of anatomical knowledge must have been a handicap in the reduction of fractures in prehistoric times, although I think primitive man was most probably familiar with the splinting method. In fact, as Sigerist (1951) emphasises, this treatment, like so many others, must have been invented spontaneously in various parts of the world: for thousands of years, people with healed broken legs must have limped forever once the leg had become inches shorter, until someone had the bright idea to stretch the broken leg to its normal length; then he found out that the leg had to be kept stretched in order to remain in the desired position, so he got a piece of hard material such as bark, attached it to the leg and the now splinted fracture healed without shortening.

The study of modern primitive societies supports the fact that treatment of fractures by reduction and splinting is a simple and logical knowledge to acquire, since the victim otherwise feels pain, and there is no reason to suggest that this was not the case in past communities (Haeger, 1988; Roberts and Manchester, 1997). The problem is that splints made from natural products, such as those identified in primitive communities today, are rarely preserved in the archaeological record.

Some examples of splints have nonetheless been identified in prehistoric Egyptian mummies, while two other sets of splints were found attached to bodies retrieved from rock-cut tombs dating back to c. 2,400 BC. The first was applied to a comminuted fracture of the middle of the femur of a young girl. The set comprised four wooden splints extended from just above the fracture to well below the knee and padded with linen bandages, the whole being bandaged in place and secured with a reef knot. There was no evidence of healing before the death of the patient. The second set was applied to a compound fracture of the radius and ulna, and comprised three pieces of bark again wrapped in linen and bandaged to the arm.

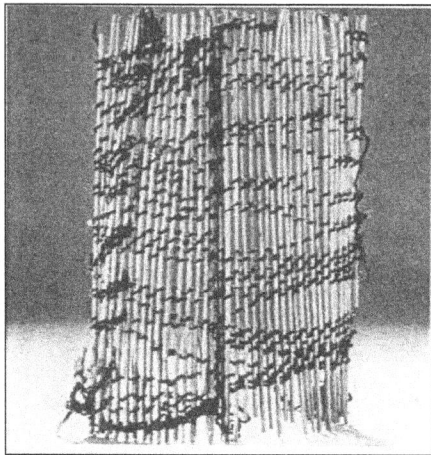

Figure 3 – Reed splint used in modern primitive societies to stabilise fractures once reduced

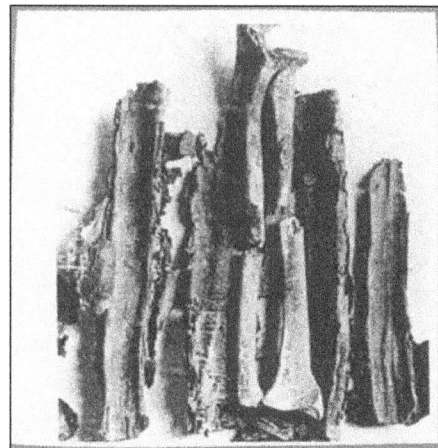

Figure 4 – Tree bark used as a splint on a mummified arm in Egypt 5,000 years ago

The wound appeared to have been plugged with vegetable fibre, presumably to staunch bleeding, but death had occurred before there was any sign of union between the bones (Sigerist, 1951; Filer, 1995).

An account of the incidence of fractures in the cemeteries at Aswan, where 6000 bodies in burials ranging from 4000 BC to the first century AD were found, shows us that results of treatment were highly variable. In some cases concerning all six long bones of the limbs, the alignment was so perfect it was barely possible to discern the fracture lines, which is particularly impressive in the case of oblique fractures of the femur, in which the pull of powerful muscles would have produced a tendency for the fragments to over ride - it is not clear how the ancient Egyptians would have arranged to sustained traction to prevent this. Most other results were far less satisfactory and there were many instances of gross shortening and malalignment (Nunn, 1996).

All over the world different cultures developed some very clever methods of immobilising a fractured limb. North American Indians set fractures with great care; dislocations are reduced by the simple medium of force and splints of cedar are applied, padded with leaves or grass and then bound with pliable branches of birch. An interesting achievement in fracture treatment is the use of form-fitting splints: the Shoshone Indians make a splint of fresh rawhide that has been soaked in water; this can be adjusted very accurately and when it dries it makes an effective cast. Other tribes use strips of bark or wood in a similar way. If the fracture was a compound one, a window could be cut into the cast to allow drainage (Vogel, 1970).

The introduction of plaster of Paris is said to have been forestalled by the natives of southern Australia, who after setting a limb encase it in clay, which hardens when dry and protects the fracture from displacement (Sigerist, 1951). Other Australian tribes simply apply slats of wood fastened by thongs, bark bound with vegetable strings, or sticks tied tightly with possum or kangaroo skins (Bishop, 1960). In the Northwest part of the country, Aborigines use human arm bones to splint arm fractures and leg bones for supporting a fractured lower limb. Rhodes (1985) reports that in the 1970's an aborigine was partially buried in sand to immobilise a broken thigh. A wide variety of fractured long bones found along the Murray River Valley, Western Australia, comprise a very interesting case. One of them was a femur with a triple comminuted fracture of the proximal half of the diaphysis; the shaft has been completely smashed and remodelled leaving it badly disfigured. What is amazing is that the bone has healed completely.

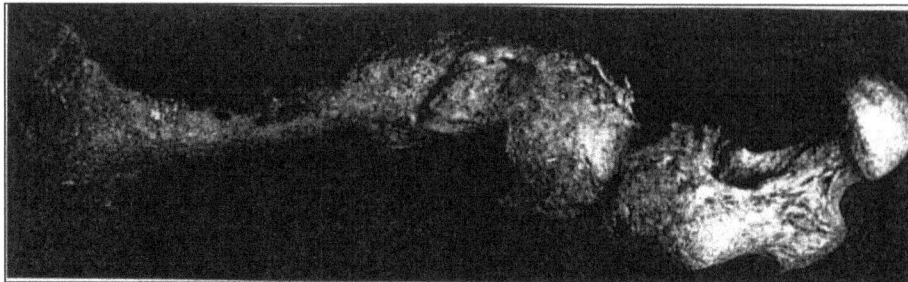

Figure 5 – A triple comminuted fracture of the femur from the central Murray, Australia

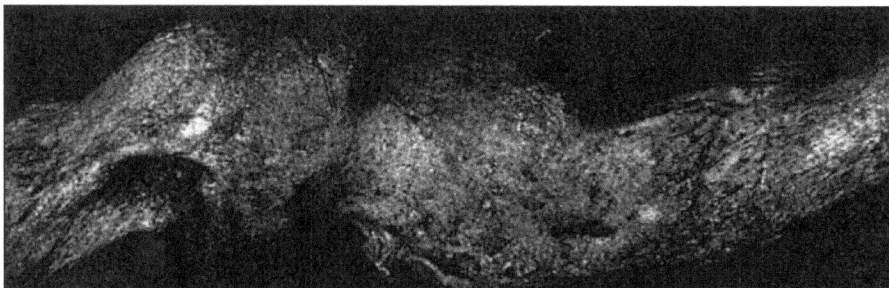

Figure 6 – Strong and large callus has developed along the fracture. There is no obvious sign of infection but substantial distortion of the shaft has taken place

It is also interesting to stress the fact that there seem to be few activities that could produce such multiple fractures (nowadays seen as the result of severe violence such as a road accident), while on the other hand fatal blood loss or infection are more likely to happen with this sort of trauma. Such fractures can take from six to nine months to heal, sophisticated traction being part of the initial nursing treatment. In the aged, healing may take longer than that or it may not take place at all without surgical intervention in the form of a plate or nail being inserted into the bone. For this bone to have mended in the way it has, there must have been a considerable amount of medical knowledge and surgical skill as well as long-term care for the patient (Webb, 1995).

The setting of broken bones is a procedure in which many African tribes have acquired considerable skill. Among the Mano, bonesetters treat a patient with a thigh fracture by placing him in a loft of a house allowing the affected leg to dangle free with a heavy stone attached. This is a very effective traction method and once the fracture is reduced, it is immobilised with a tight splint. In addition, the patient is encouraged to exercise the fractured leg so that the new bone can be laid down more rapidly over the fractured site (Harley, 1970). Other tribes dig a hole in the ground in which the arm or leg is buried and firmly held by the compaction of the earth. The body of the patient is then pulled until the bones are restored to their proper position.

The Yupik Eskimos treat a fracture by trying to realign the bones and wrapping the limb with a piece of tough, hardened skin which serves as a splint. The Nunamiut use manipulation and bound the injured limb in caribou hide with an additional splint, if necessary, to keep it straight. An interesting variation in the use of splints is that practised by Athapaskans, who encase fractured bones in a tubular piece of bark; after the initial phase of healing is complete, the bark is removed and replaced by a binding of pitch and cloth or skin. When the skin under the pitch begins to itch, healing is adjudged complete (Fortuine, 1985).

The absence of splints in fracture treatment is by no means rare. The Polynesian Tubnai give only medicine and recommend immobility; the Murngin use only poultices and heat; the Tanala apply heavy bandages but no splints. Among the Akamba, the treatment is associated with absolute immobilisation, the limb being fixed to the floor with pegs. According to Ackerknecht (1967), it is quite successful. The Hottentots rub the joint area with fat and vigorously move the limb up and down. In skull fractures African natives remove any piece of loose bone and bind leaves over the head (Bishop, 1960).

Massage as a therapeutic procedure seems to be almost universal, which is not surprising in view of the fact that it can be easily derived from the behaviour of sick animals (scratching, rubbing) and presupposes no technological accomplishments whatsoever (Ackerknecht, 1967).

15

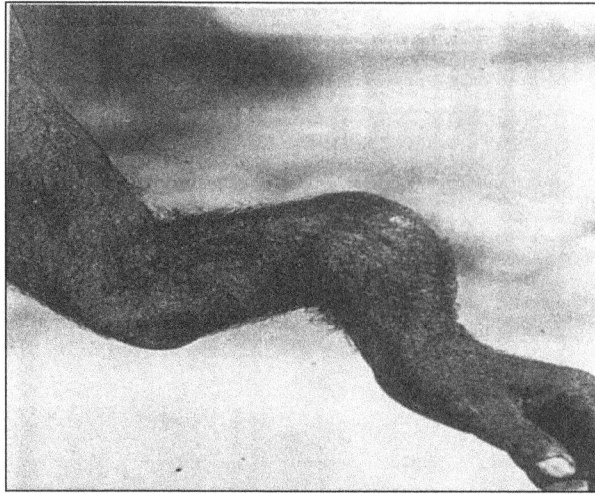

Figure 7 – No attempt was made to set the complete break of this Australian Aborigine's lower arm bones, so with the continued use the broken ends of the bones became rounded and covered with cartilage forming a ball and socket joint

4. <u>BLOODLETTING</u>

Bloodletting is the surgical removal of some of a patient's blood. Bleeding again is an almost universal trait in primitive medicine, and it can be divided into three main techniques: scarification, cupping, and venesection.

Scarification, *i.e.*, to make superficial incisions on the skin in order to produce a flow of blood, is the most widely used technique. It is reported particularly from Oceania, North America, and Brazil. In some regions it is used so freely that everybody is covered with scars resulting from the treatment (Ackerknecht, 1967). The instruments used would have varied from sharp mussel shells, flints, thorns and fish bones. Among the Dakota Indians scarification was carried out first, and then followed by suction (Bishop, 1960). The Baganda of Central Africa first scarify with a razor the exact site of operation, usually the back of the head, neck or shoulder. A small antelope or goat horn with a hole pierced at the tip is then taken and its mouth placed over the incisions. The surgeon sucks through the tip of the horn, while the blood of the patient is preventing form entering his mouth by a ward or coil of banana leaf fitted inside the horn (Bishop, 1960). In the Andaman Islands every boy and girl is scarified, sometimes for personal adornment, others as a cure for pain – for headache it is done on the forehead, for toothache on the cheek (Rogers, 1985). In South America, bloodletting was widely practiced in order to enhance the strength of the arms and legs, being performed prior to activities which required power and muscular control, while in the northern part of this continent Indians treated fevers with a liquid diet, purgation, and bloodletting (Castiglioni, 1947; Vogel, 1970). Among the Australian Aborigines of East Arnhem Land, bleeding is mainly resorted to in cases of severe headache. A deep cut is made above the brow, usually by a blow with an iron or a flint spearhead. Another method is to take a splinter of glass, and with a flick of the wrist, make a cut in the inner corner of the eye. A third technique is to split a piece of trailing cane, shape it to a sharp point, and then thrust it up one of the nostrils, which is followed by profuse bleeding (Webb, 1933).

Cupping is the act of bleeding a patient by using a container in which a partial vacuum is formed by heating. This technique is very popular in Africa, especially in the case of local hyperaemia - an excessive quantity of blood in the vessels. Outside this continent cupping is rarely found, being reported from British Columbia (Canada) and Nias (Indonesia) (Ackerknecht, 1967). Throughout Africa, cupping is practised for a wide variety of conditions, from headaches and fever to pneumonia, pleurisy, and even painful ulcers. Among the Lango of Uganda, animal horns are cut off and perforated at the blind end, wax is put over the hole and pierced to allow for suction; a few incisions are then made, whereupon the horn is put over the place and sucked until the blood flows. When the blood is flowing gently, the wax is pressed over the hole to close it, leaving the horn drawing blood. Among the native peoples of Morocco, a vein of the left arm is opened to relieve congestion of the spleen and on the right to mitigate blockings in the liver (Harley, 1970; Rogers, 1985).

Venesection or phlebotomy is the surgical opening or puncture of a vein. It is not very frequent, being mostly found in North and South America, where some Indians are said to do it by shooting a small arrow from a blowpipe into different parts of a body until a vein is pierced, which might have some magical significance. Some tribes are said to have opened veins as close as possible to the site of the pain, and in the case of severe headache, bled themselves between the eyebrows using a flint attached to a stick. (Karsten, 1926; Bishop, 1960). The Aleuts open a scalp vein with a stone lancet in instances of swelling, torpid blood, tiredness, headache, or anorexia. The Koniags also use bloodletting as a basic mode of treatment for many types of illness, while the Chugach treat sore eyes by bleeding at the root of the nose or at the temples (Fortuine, 1985).

Leeches have also been widely used for drawing blood, from a variety of locations and times immemorial – applied to every part of the body (although specially convenient for places where the knife could not be used), they would normally be left until fully gorged, then fall off.

As to the reasons for bloodletting, such a procedure is one of the most common forms of treatment for nearly everything. Many primitive cultures feel that disease is the result of bad blood and that the pain or disorder will go away if the blood is released. In Fiji a slash is made in the skin and four bamboo splinters inserted to accelerate the flow of bad fluid, while in Sumatra the blood which has been removed, considered to be the cause of illness is buried. In Ponape, any ailment that is not understood is treated by scarification and bleeding (Rogers, 1985). According to the South American Indian belief, all illnesses are caused by evil spirits which enter the system and mix in the blood. Thus, they think that by bleeding they will rid themselves of the dangerous intruder. This belief is naturally supported by the fact that in certain cases such purgation really may give some relief (Karsten, 1926). Among some Australian tribes, when a person becomes sick a healthy individual is bled on his behalf, the blood then applied over the patient's body. According to Rogers, this could be the "Stone Age antecedent of the blood donor-transfusion relationship" (1985:76).

5. <u>INCISION</u>

Incision is the act of cutting out, or the surgical removal of part or all of a structure or organ. Boils are lanced among a great variety of primitive cultures, from the Thompson Indians to the African Barundi, Akamba and Dama. The Vaitapu of Polynesia lance hydroceles - accumulation of a serous fluid in a body sac, and the Uvea cut into an inflamed testis.

Other rare operations are the opening of an empyema - collection of pus in a cavity, especially in the pleura, practised by North American Indians, and the incision of a pneumothorax, which is the presence of air in the cavity between the lungs and the chest wall in cases of pleurisy and pneumonia, by people in Uganda. The Masai cut into inflamed tonsils and practise tenotomy (cutting of a tendon), as well as the multiple piercing of goitre (swelling of the neck resulting from an enlargement of the thyroid gland); they even operate on abscesses of the liver and spleen (Ackerknecht, 1967).

Deep skin infections were widespread in all Alaska Native populations. Among the Noatak Eskimos the skin in the infected area is held in a little fold and a swift incision made at that point; particular care is necessary to avoid cutting the muscles and blood vessels, and small infections are punctured at the point where they are softest (Lucier, 1971).

The Koniags are known to perform lithotomy, or cutting to remove urethral stones, by an incision with an ordinary knife at the end of the penis. In cases of multiple spreading boils of a more superficial type, the Koniag surgeon incises the abscess with a sharp shell and sucks the pus out. If there is a deep core, however, as with a carbuncle, he uses a sharp stone lancet set in wood, and plunges it into the centre of the abscess up to the handle. Then he twists the knife about, presumably to break up the niches of pus. When the pus is reached, it is either sucked out or it drains of its own accord. The Yupik do not use anything to help the abscess come to a head, nor do they lance it, but once it drains spontaneously, arctic cotton or soft under fur of some type is applied to absorb the pus (Fortuine, 1985).

Most North American Indians apply a warm poultice of cornmeal to boils, which are lanced when ripe. Canadian Indians generally allow tumours and abscesses to suppurate without any application, but if they become inflamed and painful, plasters of bruised herbs or warm poultices are used (Vogel, 1970).

In cases of the African sleeping disease, African *Trypanosomiasis*, characterised by fever, swelling and enlargement of the lymph nodes, incisions are made in the neck of the patient and the swollen lymph nodes removed. The Thonga of South Africa make incisions in the temporal region with a razor and apply a cupping horn over them in order to treat fever (Rogers, 1985). Ackerknecht (1967) claims that he has found only one place outside Africa where surgery equals similar levels: Vaitupu (Ellice Islands), where subcutaneous lipomata, the elephantoid scrotum, tuberculous glands in the neck, old leprotic and yaw ulcers are removed successfully. It is interesting to point out that while the Africans have iron knives at their disposal, these Polynesians operate exclusively with shark teeth.

North American Zuñi Indians drained breast abscesses. Rogers (1985) mentions a case where the surgeon anaesthetised the patient with Jimson weed, *Datura stramonium*, subsequently opening the breast with a stone knife, exploring the area with his finger and removing the accumulated pus.

6. <u>AMPUTATION AND EXCISION</u>

To amputate is to cut off by a surgical operation part of the body, above all a limb, usually because of injury or disease. If today we associate the amputation of a limb with a very serious accident, as an attempt to prevent the spread of infection or with deliberate removal of a badly mutilated limb, the decision to remove even part of an arm or leg by tribal societies would have been made with even more careful consideration of alternatives. Not only is the operation itself complicated but also for the hunter-gatherer the loss of a limb must have been infinitely more of a handicap than it would be to people today with the availability of prosthetics. An active lifestyle, even among more sedentary groups, necessitated the full use of all limbs and maintenance of their proper function. Observers of the more surgery-minded tribes in Africa, America and Oceania emphasise the absence of this complicated operation, which seems most likely where nature, by freezing limbs, has already instigated the procedure. Thus, we hear of the very crude amputation of frozen fingers among the Eskimos and Chippewa of North America (Vogel, 1970). The Dama represent an isolated case of amputating crippled fingers and toes (Ackerknecht, 1967). Whether the penis amputation reported from New Guinea is of a medical nature is doubtful (Ackerknecht, 1967).

Another reason why evidence of amputation is rare in the archaeological record is probably because unhealed amputated limbs can be mistaken for post-mortem breakage of the bone. Nevertheless, amputation of limbs has been carried out since very early times and for various motives. Skeletons from prehistoric sites with limb amputations have been reported sporadically from most areas of the world (Roberts and Manchester, 1997).

Reasons discussed for amputations generally fall into one of the following three broad categories: surgical intervention, judicial punishment, or trauma. As far as the first one is concerned, a great variety of diseases may lead to the necessity of removal of more than one of the extremities; some systemic diseases such as ergotism, for example, can led to gangrene. As to judicial punishment, it was quite widespread in the Ancient World. In Egypt, for example, hand amputation was broadly practised to count prisoners and the dead. Finally, primitive weapons were certainly capable of cleanly severing a limb, and the general level of violent crime in prehistory must have been high. Evidence used to attempt to distinguish between these three possibilities comes from the morphology of the stump (amputation by sawing possibly indicates surgery, militating against an injury sustained in combat), the pattern of mutilation (in cases where more than one amputation is present on a single skeleton), and supporting background archaeological information.

One of the earliest examples of this procedure comes from an adult male found in Jerusalem (Israel) dating from c. 1,600 BC. The right hand is missing and the right radius and ulna foreshortened and fused distally.

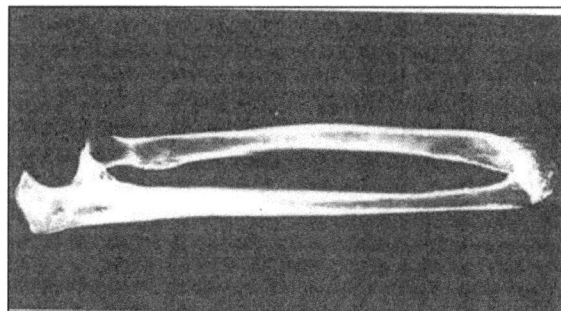

Figure 8 – Radiograph indicating full development of the radius and ulna with normal cortical thickness and firm bony union of the distal ends

The radiological appearance of this case shows healthy bone with symmetrical and complete cortical development in the amputated limbs, implying that the amputation occurred in adult life and that there was no underlying bone disease, since the bony ends were smooth with no evidence of significant periosteal reaction, bone cloacae or destruction, as would be seen if the amputation had been performed as the result of an ailment. The appearance is thus consistent with good healing without infection following surgical amputation of either a healthy hand or one traumatically damaged. In order to survive such procedure, some medical skills must have been used, which may have included precise surgical separation of the arm and wrist and subsequent haemostasis (Bloom et al., 1995).

An ancient Peruvian mummy was found with an amputated leg and a wooden prosthesis (an artificial part supplied to remedy a deficiency) which showed marks of wearing in walking attached to it (Rogers, 1985). This could possibly point towards amputation as a well planned and widely used surgical practice in Peru.

As to ethnological support, amputation for medical purposes is rare among native Africans, and usually performed with ritual implications, particularly related to mourning. A Hottentot widow who re-marries has the distal joint of her little finger amputated by tying it with sinew above the joint and then cut with a knife (Bishop, 19660). According to Ackerknecht (1967) and Magner (1992) there is only one present-day tribe, the East African Masai, that really amputates skilfully, enucleating eyes and cutting off limbs with hopelessly complicated fractures. A tight ligature is tied just above the line of amputation, the limb is placed on a hard, smooth log, and is deftly chopped off by a single stroke of a sharp sword. The Masai even have prostheses (Bishop, 1960; Harley, 1970).

The surgical technique for the pruning of a human limb is one of spectacular skill among North American Indians, since successful operations depended on speed. An amputation at the joint is performed with a knife of flint and blood vessels are sealed with stones heat until red to arrest haemorrhage (Vogel, 1970). Rogers (1985) mentions a case among the Chippewa Indians in which a man whose legs and feet had been frozen, had them both amputated. The operation was done with a common knife and the only dressing was made of bark, but the healing had been complete. The Alaska natives perform amputation when they think there is no alternative: either following a serious mutilating injury or as a sequel to frostbite. In the latter case, the gangrenous portion of the frozen limb had usually become well demarcated and anaesthetised before cutting and trimming is undertaken (Fortuine, 1985).

Webb (1995) describes two examples of amputation from the central Murray region (Australia) which involve the removal of the leg above the knee. The exact sex and age of these bones are not known, but both are from a grown adult. The first example is a left femur which has the distal one third of its shaft missing. Minor osteophytosis has formed around the stump together with patches of periostitis and osteitis.

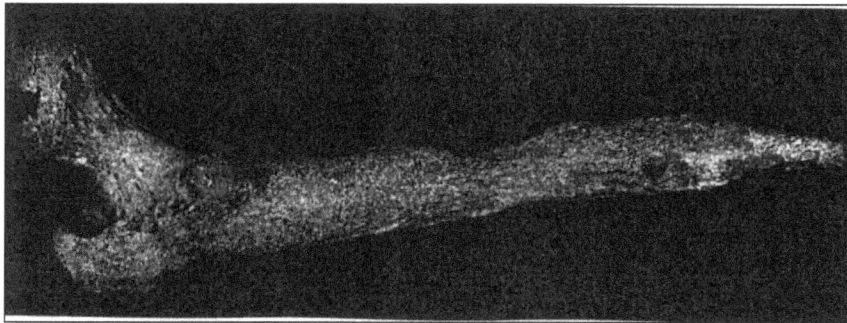

Figure 9 – Amputated femur from the central Murray (Australia) showing extensive remodelling of the bone along most of the remaining shaft

An osteomyelitic lesion lies just beyond the pencilled portion of the shaft, and the small cloaca in the bottom points to a secondary osteomyelitic infection. The second example involves a right femur. This bone has many of the features of the first, except that the amputation took place closer to the knee. Osteophytosis is present, as well as extensive osteomyelitic infection.

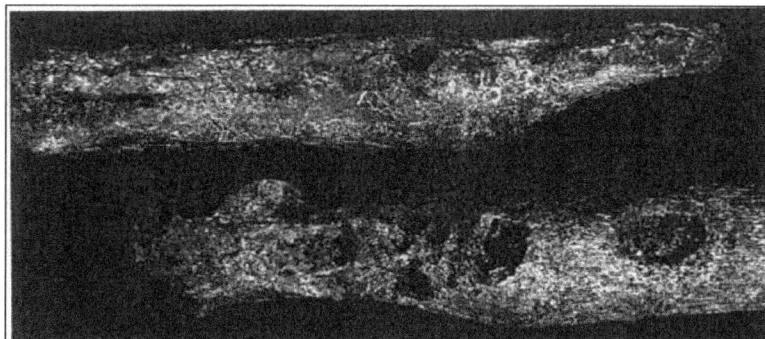

Figure 10 – These femora from central Murray (Australia) have signs of infection around their amputated stumps

Both bones are tapered to a pencil-like point at their distal ends, typical of well-documented changes that take place after this type of operation. Either the infection in these bones arose from the procedure itself, or it was a primary infection which was the reason for the amputation in the first place. In fact, some infections make the leg useless, extremely painful and a handicap, and the only remedy is amputation in order for the individual to lead any sort of active life, drastic though it sounds. Severe injury could be another reason for this surgery but there is little evidence for its occurrence in both examples. "From the general paucity of information concerning traditional Aboriginal amputation, I would assume that while this type of surgery was undertaken from time to time, it was something that it was not practised regularly and only when there was little alternative" (Webb. 1995: 216).

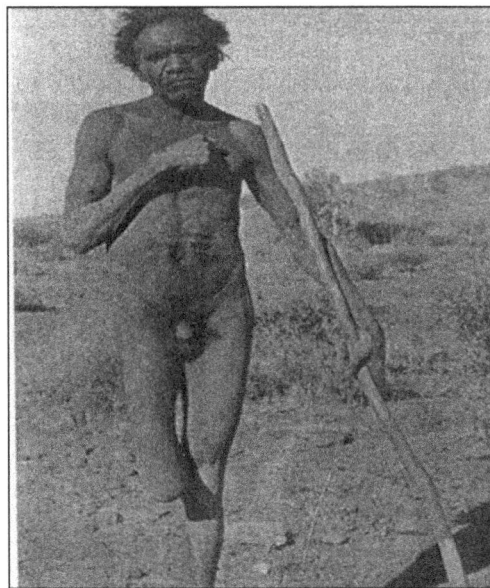

Figure 11 – Central Australian Aborigine with an amputated right leg who has taken to using a crutch

7. <u>CAESAREAN SECTION</u>

Caesarean section is the operation for delivering a child by cutting through the wall of the mother's abdomen, and it is obviously more difficult from a technical point of view than the operations mentioned above[1]. This procedure may be very old, but neither self-inflicted ripping of the belly by desperate mothers nor the widely practised cutting out of the foetus when the mother has died can qualify as surgery. While some experts dismiss reports of primitive caesareans as mere fable or misunderstanding (Ackerknecht, 1967), others stress that such an operation is one of the oldest in the history of medicine (Young, 1944).

A caesarean section was witnessed in 1879 in Uganda by a British physician who described it in great detail. The patient, a girl of 20 years of age, was given plenty of banana wine which would serve both as an anaesthetic and disinfectant, and was tied to the bed. The surgeon, assisted by two men, washed his hands and the patient's abdomen with wine, then with water. After having first pronounced an incantation he gave a shrill yell that was answered by the crowd outside, whereupon he made a quick incision from the navel to the pubis, cutting through the abdomen as well as through the uterus wall. The amniotic fluid immediately escaped and the bleeding points were touched by an assistant with a red-hot iron in order to prevent haemorrhage. The child was taken out quickly and turned over to an assistant. The cord was cut and the placenta was removed by hand. The abdominal wound was covered temporarily with a porous grass mat, and the patient was raised to let the fluid out. Then the wound was closed with seven thin nails and strings. The child was alive and the wound had healed on the eleventh day (Sigerist, 1951; Ackerknecht, 1967).

---

[1] Its name derives from the fact that the Roman law demanded that when a pregnant woman died, the child had to be removed. This caesarean regulation also stipulated that the operation could not be performed on a living pregnant woman until the tenth month of gestation.

8. <u>TREPANATION</u>

Trepanation can be defined as the practise of making a hole in the skull. The operation involves incision of the scalp, cutting through, and removal of a rectangle or disc of skull bone (roundel), the result being the exposure of the membranes covering the brain.

Considered by many the most fascinating surgical operation in the history of medicine, the bibliography on trepanation is vast but outmoded, while on the other hand there is too much controversy.

Ancient examples of trepanation number well into the thousand and their distribution is world-wide; it was practised on every continent through every period right up to our time, continuing to be practised among many modern primitive peoples. It has been reported that Mesolithic trepanned crania have been found in Russia, while other experts based on evidence from Poland, place the beginnings of this practice at the end of the Palaeolithic period. These estimates are however hypothetical, and most authors (Horsley, 1888; Parry, 1917; Piggott, 1940; Oakley *et al.*, 1959; Roberts and Manchester, 1997, between others) accept that such operation was first practised in the Neolithic. Many examples have been reported from various regions of Neolithic Europe: in particular France, Germany, Denmark, Italy, Russia, and the Balkans have revealed quite a large number of skulls. After this period, trepanned skulls become rare on this continent, but maybe this has to do with the fact that in the Bronze Age the dead were mostly cremated and thus evidence of such practise has been lost. We know that from then on trepanation continued to be performed in Europe, never reaching either the frequency nor the universality it had enjoyed in the Neolithic Age. Until the 19th century it was a conventional surgical procedure, particularly in head injuries and for various headaches and mental problems. With the spread of modern ideas about neurosurgery, the practise declined in the advanced areas of the world, continuing however to be practised until at least the beginning of the 20th century in the mountains of Serbia and Albania (Ackerknecht, 1967).

More trepanned skulls have been found in Peru and Bolivia than in all the rest of the world together. The oldest evidence dates to 3,000 BC. Trepanation was still practised by the Aymara Indians of Bolivia and was actively suggested as a cure for headache as recently as 1950. The operation was also known in Alaska, British Columbia, United States and Mexico. There are no certain reports that it is still carried out today by Indian tribes, but Margetts (1967) considers it to be possible.

Apart from Europe and South America, the evidence of prehistoric examples is quite scant, which nevertheless may be due to the fact that fewer exhumations have been carried out in these parts of the world and further excavations may reveal more information. The ethnographic evidence is however abundant.

In Asia the oldest trepanation found so far comes from Jericho, dating from c. 2,000 BC. Three Iron Age skulls have also been reported. This type of surgery was likewise performed in ancient times in the region comprising eastern Afghanistan, northern Pakistan, and Kashmir. There are in addition a couple of prehistoric examples from Siberia.

In Oceania it is still carried out by native traditional medical practitioners in the Pacific Islands of Polynesia, Melanesia, in the Loyalty Islands, Bismarck Islands, and New Caledonia.

As to Africa, a few examples have been found in Egypt, the earliest one dating from 1,200 BC. In other African countries this type of surgery has survived to the present day. We have reports from, between others, Uganda, Somalia, Ethiopia, Tanzania, Algeria, and Kenya.

As to the procedure itself, initial incision of the scalp was a very bloody procedure, but the haemorrhage can be minimised by turning back the scalp flaps created, which was certainly carried out by early surgeons. After cutting the soft tissues, the outer skull surface was exposed. At this point the pattern varied. Five different methods of trepanation have been identified from skeletal material worldwide:

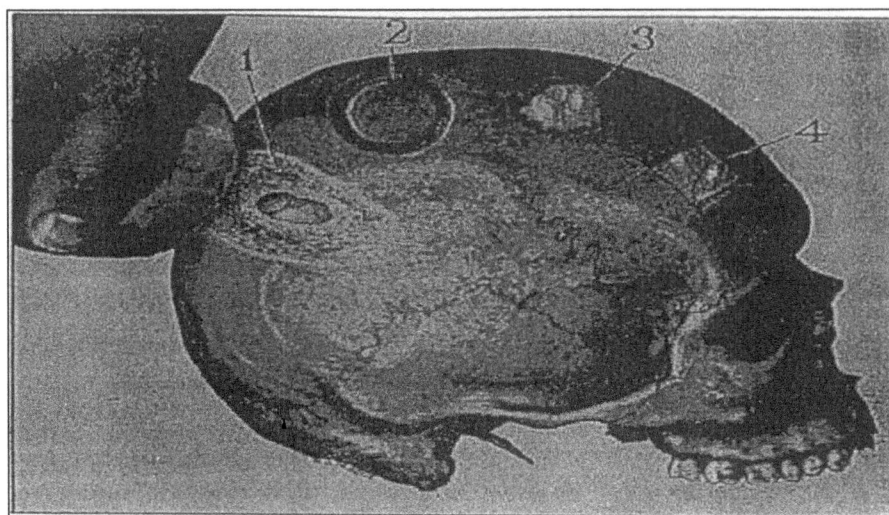

Figure 12 – Methods of trepanning: (1) scraping; (2) grooving; (3) boring and cutting; (4) intersecting incisions

The most widely used is careful scraping through the bone with a sharp implement. The resulting opening has widely bevelled edges and the removed part is in powder form. This method undoubtedly involved the lowest risk of damaging the brain, and is found in all geographic areas where trepanation occurs. Bennike (1985) reports that this was the technique used in prehistoric Denmark, all skulls in which it had been employed indicate recovery had occurred.

In the grooving method a series of curved grooves are drawn and redrawn in the skull with a sharp instrument until the bone between the grooves becomes loose and can be removed. This technique was also very frequently used in many parts of the world, such as prehistoric Romania, and it is still performed today in some parts of Africa.

In the boring-and-cutting technique the bone is pierced by a circle of closely adjoining perforations extending to the internal lamina which are then connected by cuts with a sharp instrument, the latter more or less completely obliterating the serrated border; finally, the freed fragment is levered out. This procedure was most common in Peru, also being carried out until recently among the Kabyles in Algeria.

Finally, a method in which four straight incisions are made, intersecting at right angles, and the in-between fragment is removed. This procedure seems to have been more common in Peru, but we also find it in Neolithic France, Iron Age Palestine and modern day Algeria.

The diameter of the trepanation can vary from that of a small hole of a few millimetres across to quite large openings of 82mm x 62mm or even larger. Their shapes are frequently oval, the longer diameter tending to be anteroposterior. Derums (1979) reports the case of a Neolithic skull from Latvia which possessed 3 trepanning defects in the skull, the largest single hole measuring 68mm x 55mm, and all 3 merging to produce an opening 120mm x 60mm in size. Surprisingly, the individual survived this horrific surgical trauma.

The depth of bone removal also varies: the surgeon can either remove the outer table of bone and diploë or both tables of bone, exposing the dura.

The majority of trepanned specimens show single openings, but several examples exist of individuals having undergone more than one trepanning operation.

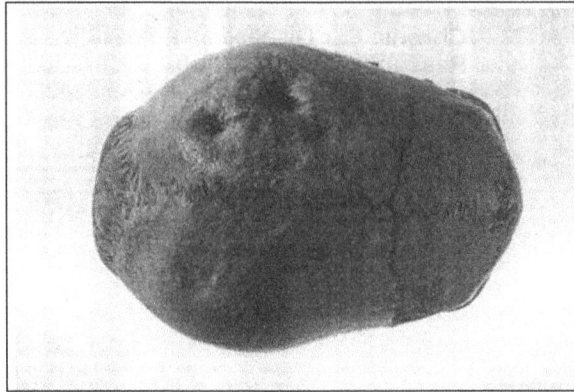

Figure 13 – Peruvian skull showing three trepanations

In Cuzco (Peru), Oakley *et al.* (1959) reported the skull with the highest number of trepanations so far discovered, showing seven healed openings. In present-day Kenya quite a number of individuals walk around having recovered from their second or even third trepanation (Margetts, 1967).

Various attempts have been made to assert the time it took to perform a trepanation. Broca (1876) experimented the operation on adult post-mortem skulls and found that it took about thirty minutes to one hour to perform it, while Lucas-Champonnière (1912), experimenting with flint instruments, needed only thirty five minutes to complete the operation (Lisowski, 1967).

Four basic responses can occur after such an operation: (1) in those cases where trauma preceded it, death may be due to the initial trauma; (2) the surgical procedure itself may cause death if there is haemorrhage or brain damage; (3) the surgical course of action may introduce disease organisms that cause infection and possibly death (sepsis, meningitis); (4) there may be no complications resulting from surgery, in which case the individual survives.

Hardly anything is known of the ancient postoperative treatment of trepanation. It is possible that prehistoric medicine-men have used powdered charcoal, hot sand, cedar wood resin or even cinders for their dressings. Hilton-Simpson (1913) reports that the Kabiles of Algeria used daily applications of heated honey and butter and stems of leaves for as long as a month. The actual trepanned opening could either be left open (possibly resulting in damage but with less risk of infection), or be covered with a durable plate or "stopper" made of materials such as gourd, shell or bone. There are a few Peruvian examples where the hole in the skull has been covered by a plaque of shell or gold (Wells, 1964). Crump (1901) states that in Melanesia the trepanned opening was washed with fluid from the unripe coconut, plugged with a piece of bark cloth and then covered with the leaf of a banana palm which had been held over a fire; then the skin flaps were replaced and stitched with a bone needle; finally the head was bound with dried strips of banana stalks. Postoperative care in prehistoric times was certainly minimal, but one thing these patients had in their favour was a minimum of contamination and infection through close association with people, since communities were small, and the use of contaminated equipment from patient to patient.

If there is no healing, as evidenced by the lack of remodelling of the cut edges or fill in of exposed, diploic spaces, the reasonable assumption is that death occurred at the time of, or shortly after surgery. A zone of porous, reactive bone surrounding the surgical area suggests survival for some time, but with the possibility of infection. Partial to complete refill of the surgical defect by remodelling of the bone around the operation site is indicative of recovery and long term survival after surgery.

The survival rate of individuals who underwent this operation was remarkably high. Stewart (1958) examined 214 trepanned skulls from Peru and found that 55.6% showed complete healing, 16.4% early stages of healing, and 28% no healing.

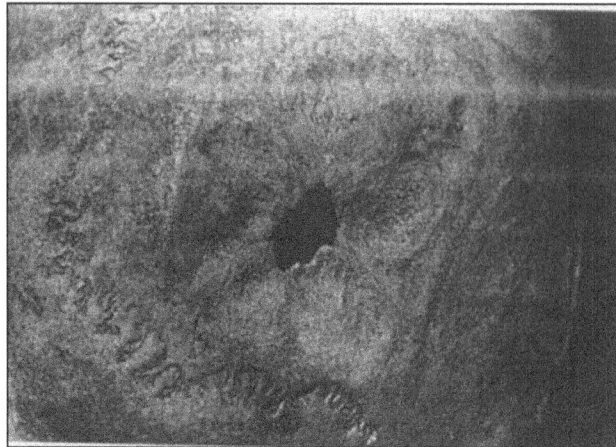

Figure 14 – Peruvian skull showing healed trepanation – the opening shows smooth borders and a closed diplöe

In a study of Neolithic material in Germany, Lisowski (1967) reports that thirteen patients survived and only three died. Bennike (1985) also observes from Prehistoric Denmark that a remarkably large proportion – 79% of the trepanned skulls – show signs that the persons have recovered from the intervention, entire or partial healing of the wound edges having occurred.

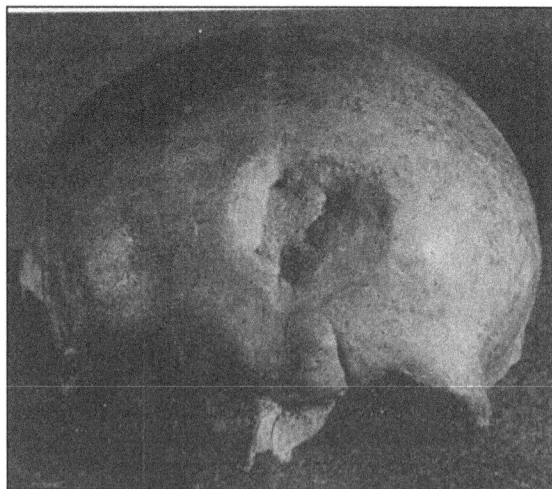

Figure 15 – Healed trepanation almost in the centre of the frontal bone of a Neolithic Danish skull

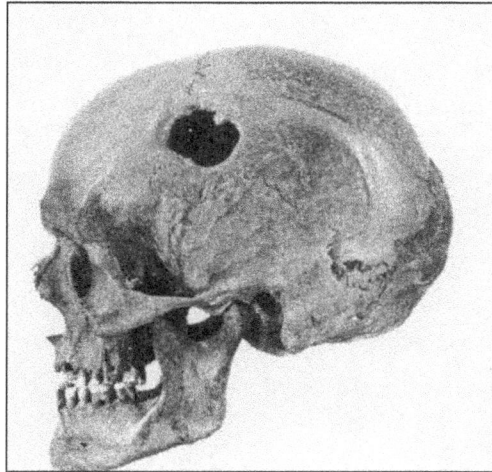

Figure 16 – Partially healed trepanation on the coronal suture between the left parietal bone and the frontal bone of an Iron Age Danish skull

There is much difficulty in identifying a trepanation in an archaeological specimen, mainly because there is a high number of different conditions that may produce similar holes. Thus, some of the so-called examples of trepanation may be cases of dysraphism, tuberculosis, syphilis, localised osteomyelitis, mycoses, dermoid cysts or myelomas.

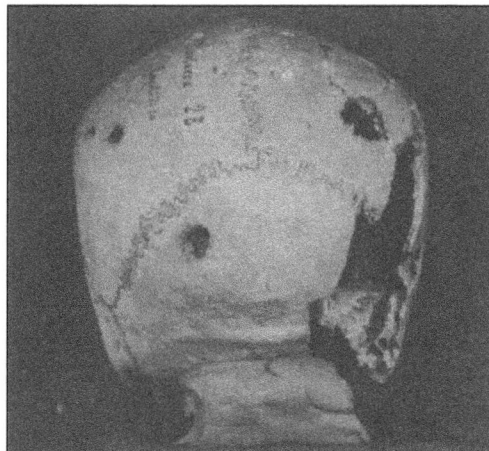

Figure 17 – Neolithic skull from the Pyrenees displaying perforations caused by a multiple myeloma

Injury can also remove a portion of the skull and produce a similar lesion, as well as the action of some rodents, beetles or porcupines (Alt *et al.*, 1997). Finally, a trephine-like wound may not have been part of a surgical procedure on the living; some groups practised post-mortem removal of circular pieces of skull (Manchester and Roberts, 1997).

In most ancient cases the motive for trepanation is not known for certain. The pain involved and especially the threat to life inherent to the procedure raise questions regarding the motives for undertaking this dangerous operation. The archaeological evidence suggests that in many cases trepanation was a surgical procedure associated with head injuries. In Danish skulls it is found almost exclusively in male specimens, with the left side being the one most commonly operated on. Bennike (1985) suggests that this pattern indicates this was the therapeutic procedure for a blow to the cranium resulting from violence among men and inflicted by a right-handed opponent. In view of the Peruvian evidence, Stewart (1958) also states that trepanations were mainly performed in cases of skull fracture, although the author does not exclude other motives for the treatment.

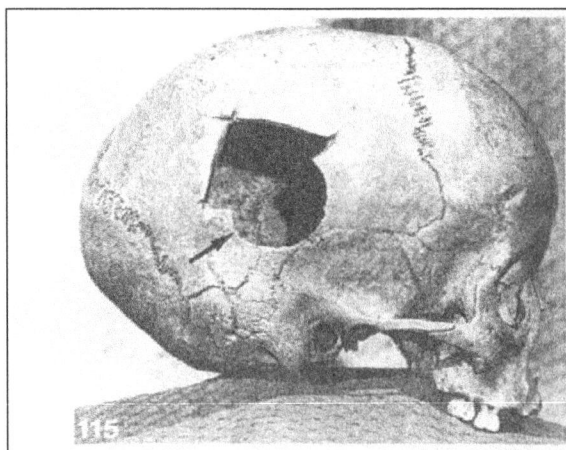

Figure 18 – Trepanation by cutting on a child from Peru. There is clear evidence of association with trauma - long circular fracture and radiating fracture extending from the former. There is no evidence of healing

36

However, in my opinion this procedure was such a frequent custom among the inhabitants of Peru and Bolivia that it might have bordered on to a cult - in this case the surgical indications must have been both therapeutic and superstitious. Effectively, in prehistoric times most diseases were ascribed to evil spirits and therefore the cure was obtained by letting these out of the skull.

As Oakley *et al.* (1959) remarked, so many trepanned skulls have been found in the chambered tombs of the Seine-Oise-Marne area of France that it is probable that the operation had some ritual significance. However, it is hardly credible that trepanation had been carried out solely for magico-ritual reasons. On the other extreme, Horsley (1888) considered that all of these operations were therapeutic, which is also far from credible. Piggott (1940), among others, considers that these interferences were performed either to repair a fracture of the skull or to alleviate headache.

Ethnographic evidence seems to stress both the religious-ritual and the medical aspect of the procedure. In many primitive psychologies, the head is the dwelling place of the intellect and of the soul, and being so it is reasonable to think of a hole in the head as an exit for an inhabiting foreign spirit. As late as the 19th century, trepanations were performed in Serbia and Albania in cases of both mental diseases and skull trauma. Brothwell (1981) points out that in New Ireland the operation had become fashionable with no other reason than that it was considered to be an aid to longevity, the same reason being given in Melanesia (Crump, 1901). In Algeria trepanation is indicated in certain cases of head injury, usually a fracture resulting from blows from sticks or stones, but the procedure is more often performed in cases of persistent headache (Hilton-Simpson, 1913). Oakley *et al.* (1959) report that in Bolivia trepanation is still performed for head injuries, while according to Margetts, (1967), in present-day Kenya the most common motive is headache.

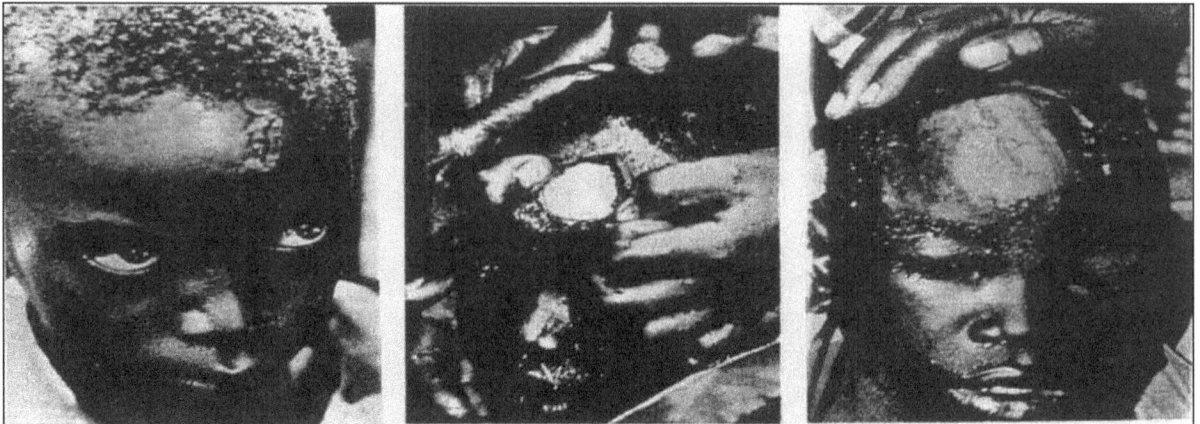

Figure 19 – Photographs from a video showing a trepanation of an African child after injury to the frontal region: (a) the patient prior to trepanation; (b) the patient with the skull exposed during trepanation; (c) the patient post-trepanation with bandages

Lisowski (1967) claims that in the Southern Pacific the surgery was used in cranial injuries due to warfare, and in some young children women cut openings into their foreheads to ward off future troubles from trauma, *i.e.*, an extension of surgical therapy to prophylaxis.

One of the many prehistoric examples of individuals who underwent trepanation during their lives was found in the Bronze Age site of Canaanite (Israel). The interesting fact of this case is that the trepanation has been made in a child of 8-9 years old, a very rare find in the archaeological record. Also, it is suggested that the operation had a particular therapeutic motive related to infantile scurvy, condition suggested by the pathological changes appearing in the maxilla, mandible and orbits of the specimen (Mogle and Zias, 1995). The trepanation has an elliptical shape, measuring 4.2 x 2.9 cm, and it is situated on the bregma, involving both parietals and the frontal bone.

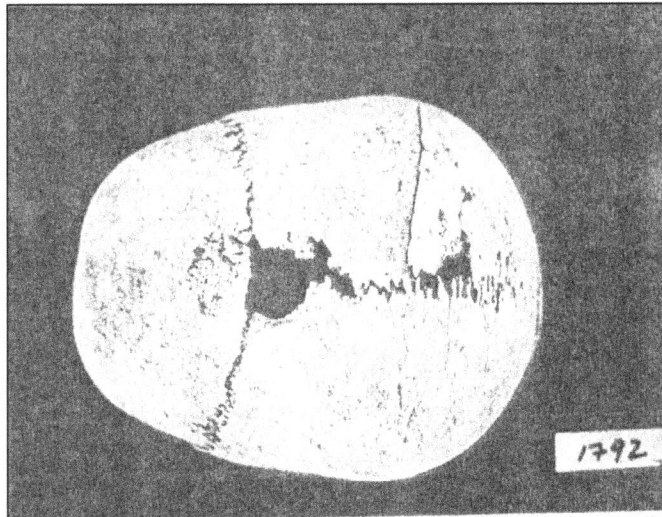

Figure 20 – Superior view of the cranium exhibiting oval trepanation

The procedure seems to have been incomplete where the lesion on the frontal bone does not penetrate the inner table, only the outer cortex and diploeic bone having been removed. The left parietal shows a bevelled circular lesion, which suggests that the technique used was the scraping one (the most common reported in the Near East). As to the mandible, it is completely edentulous, which suggests an inflammatory reactive process. "Certain metabolic problems (...) can result in inflammatory conditions that affect the soft tissues of the mouth. One such pathological process is that found in scurvy. On the skull, subperiosteal haemorrhages commonly occur on the frontal bone, particularly the orbital roof as well as the maxilla and mandible. (...) These changes are exemplified by porotic changes in the orbital roof, which are observable in the specimen discussed here (...). Advanced forms of the metabolic disturbance [scurvy] leads to bleeding from the nose and severe subperiosteal haemorrhaging" (Mogle and Zias, 1995: 79-80). According to these authors, this condition may have led to the trepanation as a form of bloodletting in hopes of draining and alleviating the consequences of this problem, which would have been interpreted as an excess of blood. The location of the trepanation on the sagittal sinus would be ideal for bloodletting. The lack of any postoperative osseous change surrounding the defect is clear evidence that the child did not survive for long, probably due to the surgical intervention itself (placed at the

39

bregma, the risk of haemorrhage of the sagittal sinus and meningeal arteries was extremely high).

A Neolithic burial of a badly mutilated and trepanned male of 25-30 years of age was found at Maiden Castle, England. On the left parietal bone several cuts have been made with the possible intent of obtaining a roundel of bone. Both the frontal and the base of the skull exhibit wounds and cuts, and in addition there are extensive injuries to the post-cranial skeleton. It is believed that trepanation has been made with the intention of removing the brain, following damage to the rest of the skull when it was found that such a procedure was insufficient to complete the objective. This case is considered to be the most convincing evidence of ritual behaviour connected with trepanning. The most plausible theory as to the likely significance of these roundels was that they were thought to possess supernatural properties and were used to protect against evil forces or magnetize positive influences (Rogers, 1985). The practise of removing the brain has parallels in other cultures (Parker *et al.*, 1986). There is of course the question of whether the roundels had been removed from living people who had undergone a trepanation or taken shortly after someone's death. It is impossible to answer to this quandary given that premortem and early post-mortem trephine markings are impossible to differentiate.

As to ethnographic contemporary cases, I have chosen the Kisii tribe of Kenya, which still carries out trepanation primarily for the complaint of headache after an injury to the head. The operation is simple but painstaking and takes one to four hours. The medicine-men learn their work from a non-relative or from their fathers, and only men can do it. Before the operation, the surgeon prays or performs other magical procedures, but there is no set ritual. The patient's head may or may not be shaved and washed, and he is then placed on a sitting or lying position and restrained. Usually, he lies on a bed of leaves with a small log under his head. Margetts (1967: 683) reports that in one case the operator "preferred to have his patient lie on a small European style bed with his head over the edge, then to sandwich him by placing another bed upside down on top of him with a relative sitting at each corner of it!"

The scalp is incised in a linear or cruciate manner over the site of the headache and the flaps are retracted by the fingers of assistants. Sometimes an unidentified medicine is sprinkled in the site to assuage pain and charcoal or local pressure is applied for haemostasis. Any fragments of bone, foreign bodies or clotted blood are removed, and any discoloured bone or fracture line is removed by scraping the skull. The scraping is usually continued until the inner table is pierced and the brain membranes exposed. The trepan is a sharp knife with a curved tip, in order to avoid puncturing the dura and brain; less frequently, a saw is employed.

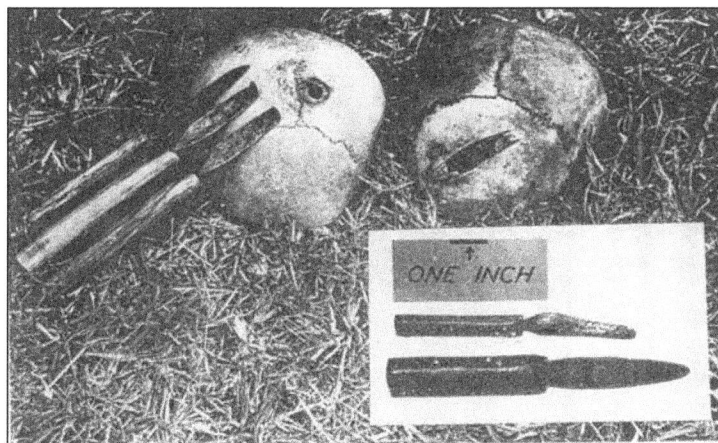

Figure 21 – Two Kenyan skulls trepanned in life with two knives, two scrapers with curved tips, and one saw. The skull on the left has been holed by scraping, the one on the right by sawing

After sufficient bone has been removed, the wound is washed with water, and fat, butter, or herbal medicines may then be applied in order to promote healing. Anaesthesia is not employed in the operation. The medicine-man watches the patient carefully during the postoperative period until good prognosis is assured. It is not uncommon for a patient to have multiple operations. As to the fee paid, it varies according to the circumstances. The mortality rate is about 5%. These patients were surely not masochistic; they really believed in some sort of a magical cure and were secure in their hope that the complaint would be relieved.

41

There is a spectacular case known as "Hat on, Hat off". This individual was about fifty years old in 1940. One day he hit his head on a door lintel while entering a hut and developed vertex headaches. He then had a trepanation, and over the next seven or eight years had several more (the exact number is unknown). He said the operations were very painful, nothing having been given to assuage pain, and the trepan used was a curved scraper.

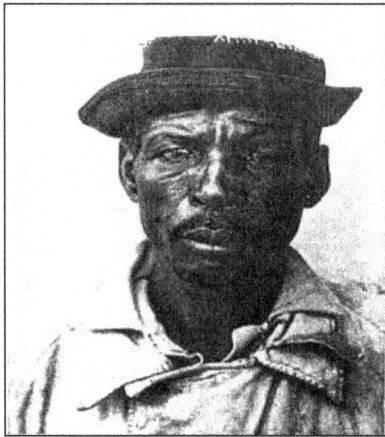

Figure 22 – "Hat On"

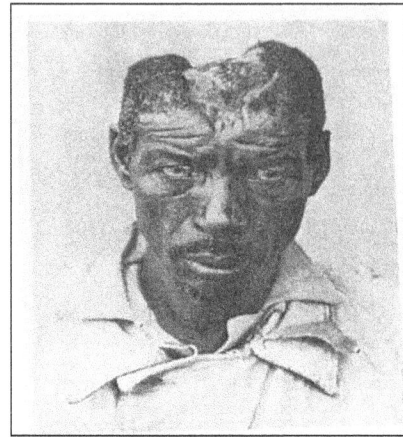

Figure 23 – "Hat Off"

He had to wear a plastic skull-cap under his hat because of the extensive cranium deficit – the whole top of his head was missing; x-ray photographs revealed an oval hole about 75 cm2 in area in the vault of his skull.

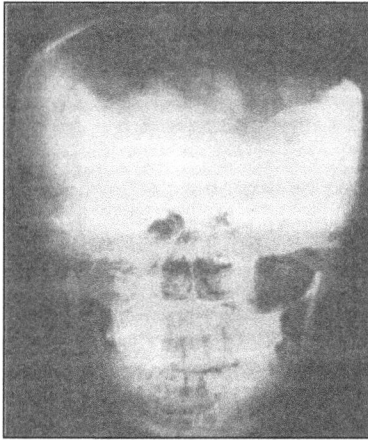

Figure 24 – Antero-posterior skull x-ray of the patient

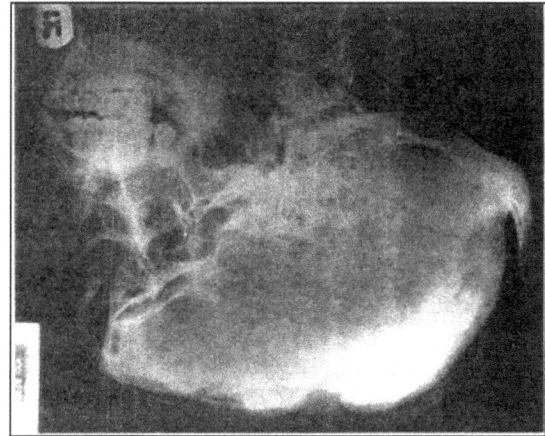

Figure 25 – Lateral skull x-ray of the patient

The surgeon who operated on him was about eighty years old, and he could not recall how many patients he had trepanned, although he claimed to have never lost a patient. His father had taught him the technique, and according to him, the only motive for trepanning was headache following a blow.

9. <u>MUTILATIONS</u>

Mutilation is the deprivation of a limb or organ, and its ritual and judicial character is widely spread in most primitive societies. Amputation of fingers for ritual reasons is well known from South and North American Indians, but the custom seems even more widespread in Africa and Oceania. For punishments, the fingers again become convenient objects if the whole hand is not sacrificed. The Seneca Indians performed a very neat amputation of half the foot upon their captives (Ackerknecht, 1967).

Next to the fingers, the genitalia seem to offer a convenient target. There are various methods of operating upon the male and female genitalia, the most common operations being circumcision and subincision.

To circumcise means to cut off the male foreskin or the female clitoris (and sometimes the labia). The origins of this most intriguing operation are lost in antiquity and have been much debated. Gairdner (1949) claims that it was originated in prehistory up to 15,000 years ago, and it was clearly sacrificial, demanding the loss of something of great value. Carvings from Stone Age France show figures which seem to have undergone either this operation or a similar mutilation, maybe for ritual purposes. If this is proved to be correct, it would be by far the earliest record of such operation (Bishop, 1960). Although it is generally believed that this operation was instituted by the Jews (who performed it as a political indicator of tribal unity and class distinction), there is evidence that the operation was carried out in Ancient Egypt.

According to some experts, this ancient operation appears to have originated in Egypt as a sign of distinction: once restricted to priesthood, circumcision was later extended to the pharaohs and their families and to children of nobility and the warrior classes (Nunn, 1996). "Eventually the operation lost part of its religious significance, and apparently the practise was enforced by hygienic reasons in all male children in Egypt"

(Rutkow, 1993:17). The idea could have been cleanliness. Especially if the foreskin is tight, it makes the tip of the penis hard to clean thoroughly. This custom was moreover a reasonable way of preventing infections under the foreskin, and the recurrence of these is treated even today by circumcision (Haeger, 1988).

Circumcision is still practised ritually among Orthodox Jews and Muslims, as well as Australian Aborigines, and various tribes in the South Pacific. In Fiji, for example, circumcision is performed as an effort to cure an ailing patient (Rogers, 1985). The operation is mainly widespread in native Africa, having gained ground mainly among the Venda and various south-eastern tribes. Among the Bambuti Pygmies of Congo, the operation is performed with significant caution and skill. Practised for initiation purposes, the young boy was carried to the back of the village and placed on a trestle. The surgeon then kneeled in front of him, holding his legs open, and performing a series of steady cuts. After about four minutes, immediately after the last cut, the wound was washed and wrapped in a leaf containing a solution prepared from roots and banana skin (Rogers, 1985). Among the Berbers of Algeria, a knobbed stick is forced against the penis glans of the patient, the foreskin being drawn over the knob and secured by a securely tied piece of string. The foreskin is then removed with a knife by a quick downward cut. Care is taken to keep demons away during operation, and after the procedure is finished, a raw egg is pressed upon the patient's penis, and juniper leaves and melted butter applied to the wound (Rogers, 1985).

This practice has also been found to prevail among a few Indian tribes in Central and South America. Among the Conibos of Peru, as soon as a girl attained a mature age, she was intoxicated by a fermented drink made of manioc roots; when she was unconscious, the operation began. An old woman cut round the *introitus vaginae* with a knife of bamboo and severed the hymen from the *labia pudendi* so that the clitoris was set quite free; some medical herbs were then rubbed into the bleeding parts and an artificial penis made of clay was introduced into the vagina of the maiden. Thereafter she was considered prepared to marry (Karsten, 1926).

Subincision is a rite which is mainly widespread in aboriginal Australia and some Pacific Islands, and generally associated with the rituals of initiation. In the male, the operation consists essentially in the slitting open of the hole or of a portion of the penile urethra along the ventral or under surface of the penis. The initial cut is generally about 2.5 cm long, but this may be subsequently enlarged as to extend from the glans to the root of the scrotum. In the female the operation takes a variety of forms ranging from extensive laceration of the vaginal walls and clitoridectomy to the slightest laceration of as much of the hymen as may still be present (Ashley-Montagu, 1936).

There has been a great deal of speculation as to the original reason for performing subincision. Among the Fijians, the Tongan islanders of Polynesia, and the natives of the Amazon basin of Brazil, subincision is carried out primarily as a therapeutic measure. Among the Fijians it is believed that it is preventive of many diseases, being also performed as a remedy following the onset of any disorder or simply to remove the evil humours of the body. The male urethra is opened and a thread is passed through so that one end hangs from the artificial opening and the other from the urinary meatus, the thread being at times drawn back and forth in order to create a discharge of blood (Rogers, 1985). Performed as a cure for tetanus among the Tongans, it is also resorted to with the purpose of removing the blood from the abdominal cavity produced by wounds in the abdomen. Among the natives of Brazil, subincision is practised for the purpose of removing the diminutive fish which sometimes gain entry into the urethra when natives bathe in the waters in which these fish abound (Ashley-Montagu, 1936).

In Australia, the operation has by many writers been regarded as a practise devised in order to limit the number of births – a contraceptive measure. Nevertheless, at the present time practically all observers agree that the Australian Aborigine had no such understanding of the physical relationship between intercourse and pregnancy. Another reason that has been suggested is that it was devised to ensure the maintenance of a proper balance between the food supply and the numbers of the population; however, there are vast areas in Australia which are well capable of supporting a much larger proportion of individuals than are ever found in such territories (Ashley-Montagu, 1936). Yet another widespread theory is that subincision is a male counterpart of female menstruation that clears the male of toxic constituents through an artificial opening that is anatomically analogous to the female vulva. Finally, it has also been cited as a means of bloodletting for therapeutic purposes.

I think it is reasonable to state that the operation must have undergone divergent lines of evolution which have greatly modified its original purpose. The element that is undeniably common to all forms of subincision is the effusion of blood, which leads most scientists into thinking that male subincision is intended to correspond to female menstruation: menstrual blood is a noxious humour, and judging this to be the natural manner of getting rid of the bad humours of the body, they essayed to produce an artificial menstruation within the males' bodies. Women are cleansed by the process of menstruation, but men, in order to guard against disease, have periodically to incise the penis and allow a quantity of blood to flow. Thus, the operation here is of a prophylactic nature, but it is at the same time a strongly magico-religious procedure (Ashley-Montagu, 1936).

A Neolithic mutilation of difficult interpretation is the so-called sincipital T. Such procedure was first found on a number of female skulls from ossuaries of the Seine-et-Oise, France, and consisted of a T-shaped scar beginning on the frontal bone, running all along the sagittal suture, and branching into two parts along the posterior edge of the parietal bones.

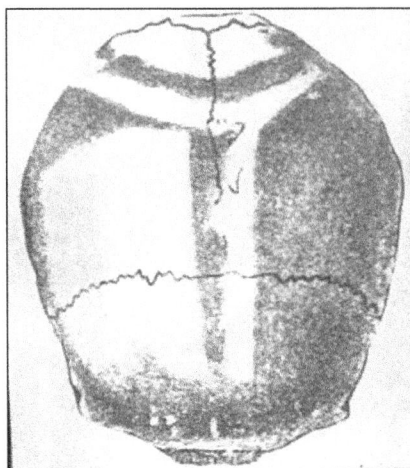

Figure 26 – Sincipital T scar

The scars may have been caused by deep incisions through the scalp or most probably by cauterisation. While the T-shape was the rule, a few skulls were found with a straight line or oval cicatrices (Magner, 1992; Ortner and Putschar, 1981). Prehistoric skulls with the same peculiar lesion have been found in Peru and India. We have no way of ascertaining the reason why this obviously painful operation was performed, whether it was for therapeutic, magical, religious, judicial or cosmetic ends, or as a punishment. Nonetheless, the prevailing opinion is that this was done as a cure for headache, melancholia, epilepsy, and other nervous conditions that involved convulsions (Rogers, 1985). In Medieval times the scalp was cauterised by Arabic physicians in the treatment of various nervous diseases, while deep scarifications of the forehead were practised by Alexandrian surgeons in the treatment of eye ailments.

Oval scars similar to one from Seine-et-Oise were found on the skulls of the Guanches, early inhabitants of the Canary Islands, who made large scarifications with stone knives on the part affected and then cauterized the wound with roots of malacca cane dipped in boiling grease (Sigerist, 1951; Bishop, 1960).

However, we also have to bear in mind that evidence for this procedure could, in fact, have originated from something else. There is for example the possibility of senile athrophy, which can occur in the sagittal and lambdoid sutures, producing a

48

depression very similar to the changes reported for sincipital T mutilation. A prehistoric skull from Georgia (USA), appearing to be that of a female over 50 years of age, exhibits a depression in the posterior sagittal suture and much of the lambdoid suture; there is evidence of senile atrophy medial to both temporal lines (Ortner and Putschar, 1981).

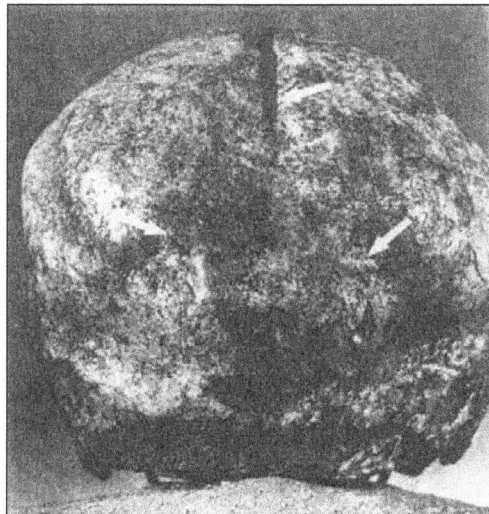

Figure 27 – Atrophy of the skull in the region of sagittal and lambdoid sutures

These are all interesting analogies and, while it is possible that Neolithic man did perform these T-shaped cuts for similar reasons, we can not do more than speculate about it. It is interesting to point out that most of the French victims of this operation were females, which might mean that the procedure had a ritualistic or punitive function rather than a therapeutic purpose.

10. TEETH

Due to their hard and robust structure, teeth are often the only part of the body that survives to be excavated by archaeologists. Nevertheless, evidence of dental surgery has rarely been reported. The biggest problem here is to differentiate between ante-mortem tooth-loss and deliberate extraction.

Roberts and Manchester (1997) report an individual from Israel, dated to 200 BC, with a 2.5 mm bronze wire implanted in a tooth, as well as a Danish skeleton dated from the Neolithic which has a drilled cavity between the roots of the first and second upper molars. Even though dental surgery seems to have been very rare in Ancient Egypt, one case of apparent significance has been found in Giza in a specimen which dates from around 1,500 BC. – a mandible with two round 2.5 mm holes bored in it, apparently with the intention of draining an abscess below the first molar on the right side. They had been placed with skill so as not to impinge on the roots of the teeth and are said to be the oldest example of oral surgery on record.

Bennike and Fredebo (1986) account a case found in a passage grave in Langeland, Denmark, dating back to c. 2500 BC. This was the skull of an adult male with a molar in which it looked like a hole had been drilled. The circular cavity has a maximum diameter of 4 mm and a depth of 6 mm. Caries would have been so pronounced that it led to an infection of the soft parts and nerves of the tooth, which resulted in a chronic inflammation and root abscess manifesting itself in a round cavity. From there the drainage possibly took place through perforation of the bone as an attempt to assuage the pain. There is advanced atrophy of the tissue around the roots of the teeth, a condition we today recognise as pyorrhoea, in which the roots of the teeth are gradually exposed. But would this hole have been made while the person was living? The most telling evidence is the tartar found on the inner surface and edge of the drilled hole during the electronmicroscopic examination, meaning that the man was not only alive when they drilled into his tooth, but that he also lived for some time thereafter. "It is likely that the treatment of toothache has been attempted in other locations in prehistoric times but it is at Langland that we have the first and earliest evidence that dental treatment in the form of drilling a hole was performed in the Stone Age." (Bennike and Fredebo, 1986:86).

11. <u>CUTTING FOR THE BLADDER STONE</u>

The cutting for the bladder stone is, according to Ellis (2001: 183), "the most ancient operation taken for the relief of a specific surgical condition", performed the earliest days for reasons other than the emergency care of an injury. The oldest bladder stone we know of dates from about 4,800 BC and was found in the grave of a teenager in the cemetery of El Amrah in Egypt. Unfortunately, the specimen was destroyed when the Hunterian Museum (Royal College of Surgeons, London) was bombed during World War II.

There are three possible surgical approaches to remove a stone from the bladder: by cutting down on to the base of the bladder through the perineum, immediately in front of the rectum (perineal lithotomy), by passing crushing instruments into the bladder along the urethra (suprapubic lithotomy), and by opening the bladder thorough the lower abdomen (transurethral lithotomy).

12. MAGIC IN SURGERY

If we understand the term "medicine" as the relief of pain by our own means, or the repair of damage produced by injury or disease, we should think first of its instinctive origin. In fact, the first expressions of pain are instinctive. Examples of such a procedure are frequent even among animals: they instinctively alleviate fever in cold water, hunt the parasites that torment them, and try to lessen the pain of their wounds by licking them. Empirical medicine is soon derived from these instinctive ideas.

Early man most certainly did not admit the existence of disease from what we call natural causes. Because of pain, persevering injury and possible death, serious illness provoked agony and anxiety, being hard to accept as an accident with no meaning. He regarded his ailments as being the result of the malevolent influence exercised by supernatural beings or human enemies. Effectively, among modern primitive societies it is a common belief that malady is either caused by the loss of something essential to life or by projection of some morbid material or influence into the victim. To this extent, the prehistoric surgeon's processes were undoubtedly charged with mysticism and fostered groundings aimed at the appeasement of supernatural forces.

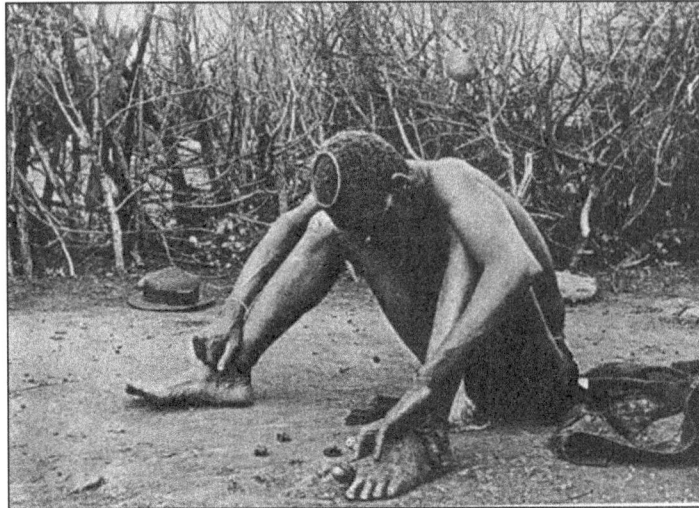

Figure 28 – Medicine-man from Zimbabwe reading the divine bones for diagnosis of the cause of illness

Furthermore, primitives do not distinguish between medicine, magic and religion. To them they are one, a whole set of practises intended to protect them against evil forces and to bring them good luck. Supernatural influences are regarded as major controlling factors in the events of daily life. Thus, they are based upon an animistic attitude towards disorders, *i.e.*, such phenomenon was caused by the evil influence of an enemy, a demon, a god or an animal who had projected an alien spirit, a stone, or a worm into the body of the unsuspecting patient. As a result, it is in empirical medicine that magic medicine has its origin: if one believes that supernatural forces are the cause of disease, it is evident that to be cured, one must combat these malignant influences with the aid of supernatural powers (Castiglioni, 1947; Magner, 1992). Such disabilities were thus warded off by incantation, dancing, charms, talismans, and other magic measures. If the evil influence managed to enter the body of its victim, either in the absence of these precautions or despite them, the body had then to be made uninhabitable to the demon by beating, torturing and starving the patient, violent vomiting induced by potions, or a hole bored in the skull (Garrison, 1929; Guthrie, 1958; Sigerist, 1951).

Australian Aborigines believed that no ailments are accidental, all being caused by either people or spirits practising sorcery. Whenever this happened, a man versed in magic was called in. To ensure success, magic and plants were often prescribed side by side.

When it comes to wounds, the Masai put a dead fly into them, while among the Banyankole the wounded can only be nursed by women without sexual relations. Heat used in the treatment of wounds has a symbolic meaning and makes the disease spirit fly away among the Yakuts of Siberia. Many North American Indians such as the Apache, Havasupai, and Creek treat wounds with magic songs (Ackerknecht, 1967).

As for fracture treatment, the plants used so frequently as internal medicaments or poultices have implications of magic power; this is reported from the Azande of Central Africa, among others. The Tarahumare Indians bind the heads of lizards around the fracture. At Nias, fractures and dislocations are preferably reduced by those born with their feet forward, and among the Zuñi by those struck by lightning. The Havasupai use splints and magic songs (Ackerknecht, 1967).

The instruments with which bleedings are carried out among South American tribes are of particular interest, because a special magical power is often ascribed to them. The Puris and the Coroados of the Amazon perform venesection on the arm by letting off from a miniature bow a small arrow with a piece of crystal attached, working as a charm (Karsten, 1926).

I would like to stress that it would be wrong to dismiss magic as irrelevant to the healing process. Suggestion and expectation of cure have a curative value, particularly in the relief of pain, a phenomenon now known as the placebo effect. Since in ancient times there may have been few pharmacologically effective remedies, it was entirely reasonable to rely on the placebo effect which, for many conditions, would have been much better than nothing.

13. MEDICINE- MAN

The medicine-man holds in primitive society a much more important position than a physician does in a modern community: he is priest, sorcerer and physician in one, and very often the chief of the tribe.

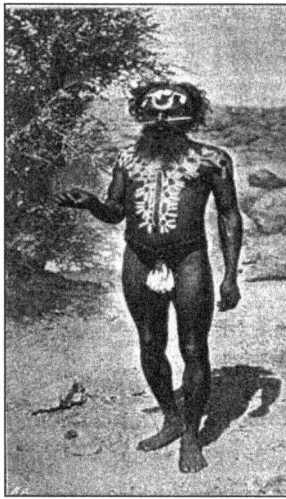

Figure 29 – Central Australian medicine-man

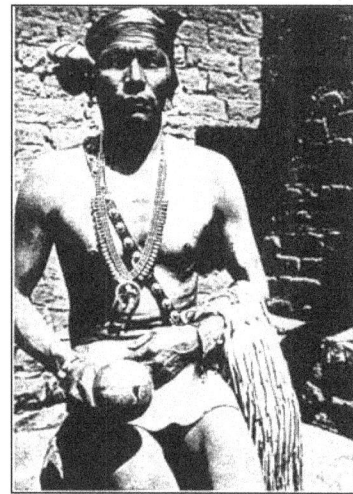

Figure 30 – Navajo medicine-man

In North America, the profession is open to both sexes but many more men enter it than women. Transmission of power by inheritance is exceptional, and in most tribes the medicine-man selects his successor, a bright young boy that he trains and uses as an assistant for many years until he becomes an independent and powerful medicine-man himself. The social position of the Indian medicine-man has always been a very high one; he is greatly respected because he is skilful and by far the best-informed man of the group (Sigerist, 1951).

The Siberian shaman has a completely different life and behaviour. The mentally ill are chosen for such chore and believed to be possessed by spirits. Shamanism is sometimes hereditary, but often a dead shaman selects his successor, who is informed of his vocation in a dream. The individuals chosen are people of a special type, dreamers, highly nervous and excitable people. They are sick and recover by shamanising (Ackerknecht, 1943; Sigerist, 1951).

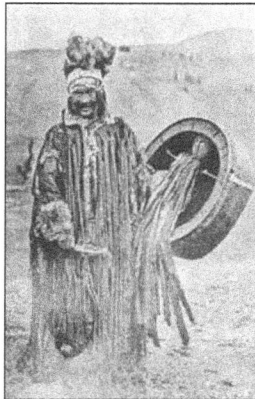

Figure 31 – Siberian medicine-man

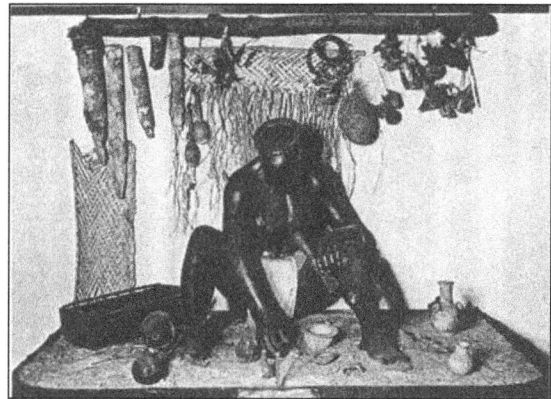

Figure 32 – Nigerian medicine-man

A medicine-man similar to the Siberian shaman is found in South Africa, particularly among the Bantu. He too is possessed by a spirit, instructed in dances and songs, in throwing the bones, in the use of drugs, in finding hidden things, and invested with protective amulets. Women are called just as men, and in some tribes more frequently than men. In other sections of Africa the medicine-man is generally of the non-inspirational type: he is trained in the knowledge of herbs, in the art of magic and in religious rituals by another medicine-man, usually his father, because a medicine-man has the desire to pass his knowledge and power to the most intelligent of his children. The profession, however, need not be hereditary, and children born under unusual circumstances or others who had strange experiences, such as falling from a tree without being injured, were often considered predestined for the task (Sigerist, 1951).

In the Alaskan native cultures the people who perform surgery include skilled practitioners (persons who had developed special skills, either through experience or through a kind of apprenticeship training), shamans (who were likely to be called in situations where surgery had failed and the case seemed desperate, their contribution being limited to magic), a close relative, or even a random member of the community (Fortuine, 1985).

In Aboriginal Australia the medicine-men are usually selected and initiated in a dream by a ghost. The medicine-man is paid for his labours, the fee being usually determined by the success of the treatment and by the social status and wealth of the patient (Sigerist, 1951).

Medical specialisation is by no means a late phenomenon of civilisation but is very frequently encountered among primitives. Its characteristics are however considerably different, *i.e.*, specialisation is one of power and function. Thus, the Havasupai have three types of medicine-man, one who has power over the weather, one who cures diseases, and one who treats wounds, fractures and snake bites (Sigerist, 1951). The Zuñi have a separate clan of bonesetters (mostly people struck by lightning), as well as the Azande, Gio and Mano. In populous tribes medicine-men are often organised in societies which have special functions: in North America the members of the Omaha Buffalo Society are specialised in surgical work (Sigerist, 1951). Only among the Masai we hear of a definite class of surgeons (Ackerknecht, 1967).

As we have seen in this brief summary, different as the medicine-men are in various sections of the world, they have nevertheless many traits in common. They are learned men, although the content of their learning is very different from what we should expect a physician to know (their physiological and anatomical knowledge is quite poor), and they perform a very important function in a society of which they are some of the most prominent members.

As to the status of the sick man, when an individual has a minor ailment, he is treated with domestic remedies and is not prevented from sharing in the life of the group. Things are different in the case of a serious illness or accident; such an occurrence gives the sick man a special position in society, not only because of the physical condition in which the patient finds himself but also the attitude of primitive societies towards the disease phenomenon. The sick man is weak and helpless, he cannot attend to his accustomed occupations, depends on others, and is a burden. Two basic attitudes towards him are observed among these peoples. Some accept the burden, treat him kindly, feed him, attend to him, and are prepared to bring any sacrifice to have him treated - Cheyenne women are willing to sacrifice a finger for the recovery of a sick family member. Others, however, get rid of the handicapped - before the sick lose too much flesh, the cannibal Bobos of Sudan kill them and eat them (Sigerist, 1951).

14. <u>ANAESTHETICS</u>

Our prehistoric ancestors probably had a greater tolerance of pain than we do. We do not know if any primitive form of anaesthesia was available, but it is more than likely that prehistoric surgeons had at their disposal various herbs and plant extracts that would have decreased pain.

As to modern primitives, the extensive knowledge of drugs they possess is astonishing. There is hardly a tribe that does not use at least some medicinal plants, and more highly developed peoples may well apply hundreds of them in the treatment of disease. Both pain and efforts to alleviate it have in fact been constant in human history, and we owe many effective drugs to primitive and folk medicine, such as opium, coca, caffeine, cinchona, ephedrine, cascara sagrada, chaulmoogra, digitalis, ipecacuanha, podophyllum, pyrethrum and squill, to mention only a few (Guthrie, 1958).

The discovery of these remedies must have been a very gradual process. Just as cats and dogs eat grasses as their medicines, so did primitive man discover the therapeutic value of certain plants. Opium poppy seeds have been found in Swiss lake dwellings of the 4th millennium BC, and opium was in use in Egypt in the 2nd millennium BC. In the 19th century it was still recommended for amputations (McGrew, 1985).

Some narcotic plants such as the mushroom fly-agaric employed in Siberia to produce ecstasy and temporary derangement of the senses during the course of ritual ceremonies could have been used as medical sedatives if properly prescribed and administrated.

There is numerous guesswork as to what degree the Peruvians may have used drugs as narcotics for producing anaesthesia in trepanation, some scholars suggesting the use of coca and peyote. In more recent times, it has been recorded that these people have treated wounds prior to surgery with powdered leaves that contain c. 9% of cocaine, hence nullifying the pain that would result from the operation. It has been suggested that this technique of local anaesthesia could have been used by the ancient Peruvians, but there is no clear evidence of either this measure or such use in prehistoric times.

Perhaps the earliest painkiller was alcohol, which was discovered long ago and is produced by nearly all peoples in one form or another. Haeger (1988) lays emphasis on the amount of descriptions as to how trepanations begin in many tribes, with the patient as well as the surgeon, getting themselves drunk.

Modern primitives prepare drugs in very much the same way as we did it until the advent of the modern pharmaceutical industry. They make decoctions and sometimes infusions of leaves, bark, roots or flowers, prepare salves and ointments by mixing the powdered drug with oil or animal fats, and they produce fumes that are inhaled or to which the skin is exposed by burning dried plants. Drugs are given internally *per se* or in the form of enemas.

For anaesthetic purposes during the operation of trepanning, the Serbians use grape wine and people from Uganda use palm wine (Lisowski, 1967). The Mano of Liberia have quite an interesting substitute for a local anaesthetic during the operations of circumcision and scarification: *Tragia sp.* is rubbed on the area to be cut; this causes such a violent itching that the cutting is welcome, rather than painful (Harley, 1970). South American Indians have no anaesthetics properly so called, but the constant use of the *Eurythroxylon coca* plant creates insensibility. The plant is always applied to wounds, bruises and contusions, and it tends to deaden pain, if not to eliminate it. In this manner, the Indians unconsciously employ an anaesthetic, although they believe only in its healing qualities (Bandelier, 1904).

As to the application of drugs, the Chiricahua Apache pour the liquid through an enema tube made of elderberry wood, and after the pouring is done, they blow into the tube. The natives of Liberia and other Africans use a gourd for this purpose, inserting the stem into the rectum; the drug is administered while an incantation is sung, and it is believed that the holy words give the drug its power (Sigerist, 1951).

Unfortunately, it is not always easy to find out what the drug lore of a tribe is, because many remedies are kept secret; they are the treasured possession of a medicine-man who may have purchased the secret for much money. Even if we succeed in obtaining a native drug, we may have a handful of dried roots or leaves and may find it still difficult to identify the plant. On the other hand, as I have already stressed, many primitive remedies must be sympathetic, and are unlikely to have major therapeutic effects.

13. <u>SURGICAL INSTRUMENTS</u>

The nature of the surgeons' instruments is an important aspect of his know-how, but unfortunately the operating equipment of prehistoric man is difficult to determine, and our knowledge of what he might have used highly conjectural.

Before the manufacture of the first implements and tools approximately half a million years ago, man would have applied his hands and mouth on impulse to stop bleeding, remove thorns, complete the amputation of severed limbs, and so on. Kirkup (1995) reports that the Klatsoops of North America pinched through the umbilical cord with their fingernails. In time, surgical instruments evolved to facilitate, extend, and refine practices where fingers alone proved inadequate or unsuccessful.

The most ancient instruments were sharpened stones that served to extract various foreign bodies, to let blood, to open abscesses, and to scarify, but they also served for more serious operations, such as trepanation (Castiglioni, 1947). Speculation suggests that the first surgical instruments were borrowed from domestic, craft, and perhaps funerary items, and it is unlikely that the makers devoted themselves exclusively to any one function; this is why few instruments from the prehistoric period have been identified with certainty (Weston-Davies, 1989). In the past, a flint or metal knife used as a weapon or for butchering meat was one and the same thing, and if applied to divide the umbilical cord, scarify skin or lance a vein, these were intermittent and non-specific roles (Kirkup, 1993). Thus, the chief difficulty for the archaeologist is that unless a whole set of instruments of undeniably surgical nature is found together, it is almost impossible to decide with any degree of certainty that a knife was employed in the operating room rather than in the kitchen or by a goldsmith. As Rogers stresses, "a stone age surgeon sufficiently skilled to perform a number of exacting operations would also have been able to fabricate from wood, thorns, stone and shell, the basic apparatus that he needed in his professional activities" (1985: 9-10).

During the so-called Neolithic (c.8,000-3,000 BC) technology advanced rapidly to produce axes, knives, arrowheads, borers and scrapers of outstanding refinement, while the discovery of copper and bronze (c.4,000 BC) and of iron smelting (c.1,000 BC) revolutionised the manufacture of weapons and tools, prompting the perfection of many crafts and leading to more durable, efficient, and compact equipment (Kirkup, 1982; Rutkow, 1993).

Nevertheless, surgical instruments, of a type that prehistoric man may have used, have been identified in modern primitive cultures everywhere.

Flint has been employed by the American Cherokee and Alaskan Indians, nephrite (jade) by the Eskimos of the Bering Strait, and glass by Australian Aborigines, for operations such as scarifying, bleeding and circumcision (Kirkup, 1993). Reed, bamboo, shell, animal teeth, and bone fragments were other early substitutes for man's hands and teeth. That organic items have played a role in solving surgical instruments is evident from observations made in non-industrialised societies. The Ellice Islanders used shark's teeth to scarify, venesect and open abscesses. Certain tribes in Polynesia conduct scarification with slivers of bamboo and thorns and in North America the Cherokee Indians use blackberry thorns and dried laurel leaves to bleed by multiple scratches (Kirkup, 1993), while the Dayaks of Borneo employ sharp roots for opening abscesses (Garrison, 1929). Crump (1901) describes the instruments used for trepanation in Melanesia, where the sharp edges of shells and shark's teeth were utilised in addition to obsidian.

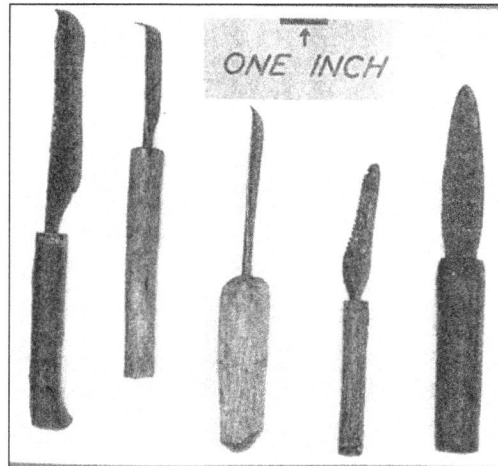

Figure 33 – Trepan instruments from Kenya

Rogers (1985) accentuates the impressive outsized number of utensils at the surgeon's disposal among the aboriginal Berber surgery. Their specialisation and variety is notable, the larger ones being made of iron with wooden handles and the smaller usually of brass and copper. Instruments were designed for particular surgical requirements. In cases of trepanation for example, there were specialised knives for cutting the scalp, drills of several types (some showing well-designed features to prevent too a deep penetration of the skull vault), assorted saws with different width teeth and a variety of small implements including retractors, elevators, hooks and forceps.

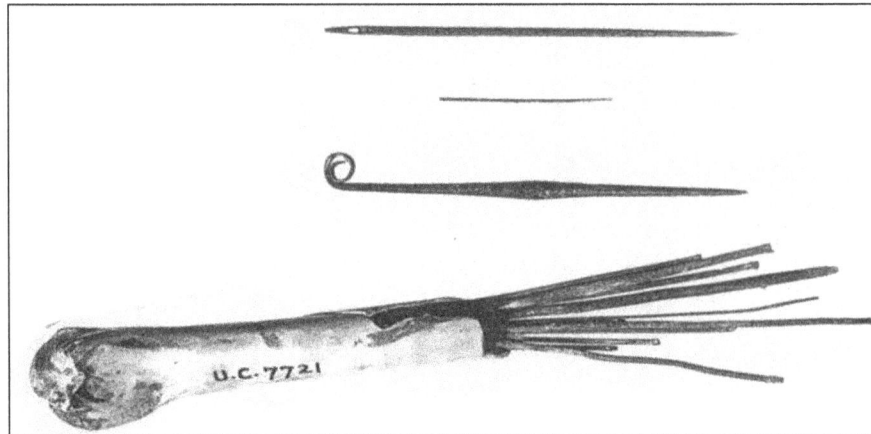

Figure 34 – Copper needle, silver needle and copper pin with loop head from Naqada, Egypt (4500-3000 BC). Below is an unprovenanced bone needle case containing fifteen copper alloy needles from Egypt (1550-1069)

Worthy of special mention is an instrument used by the Chippewa Indians for applying medicine beneath the skin and which consisted of several needles fitted into a wooden handle. According to Rogers (1985), it was used in treating dizziness, neuralgia and rheumatism, visibly representing an example of prescientific hypodermic injection.

14. DISCUSSIONS AND CONCLUSIONS

From what we have read, we can mainly distinguish between three different forms of surgery: manipulative, minor operative and major operative.

Manipulative surgery consists of the restoration of body elements that have been disturbed through dislocations or fractures without cutting of tissue. The surgeon's role in this case depends largely on his knowledge and manual skill in restoring the proper anatomical associations – he does not possess an insightful theoretical background, but shows a good understanding of skeletal anatomy. Minor operative surgery usually involves either the removal of a foreign body from the patient's body, such as a thorn or arrowhead, or the incision of boils or abscesses in order to evacuate fluid. The surgeon shows some knowledge of superficial anatomy by removing the alien object, usually by grasping, pulling and/or making an incision to reach and release the item. With regard to major operative surgery, it comprises a superior level of information and expertise, including such procedures as amputation, trepanation, and caesarean section.

From a historic perspective, surgery changed relatively little for more than 5,000 years. Some societies at different periods have proved more adept or venturesome than others, but the catalogue of possible operations before the end of the 19th century was short and dealt with the extremities while avoiding the body cavities, the central nervous system and the brain.

According to most authors, modern primitive surgery is in fact poor in scope and quality. Only in Southeast Africa and Polynesia we encounter relatively developed surgery. Even tribes with wide medicine lore, like the Liberian Manos, are extremely conservative when it comes to surgery, being basically limited to bone-setting, bloodletting and circumcision.

Theoretically, there exist five possibilities to explain why primitive surgery has not advanced further:

1 - Under primitive conditions there is no need for a more developed surgery.

2 - Primitives lack the technical skill necessary for better surgery.

3 - Primitives lack certain elements of basic knowledge, mainly anatomy, asepsis and anaesthesia.

4 - Other elements of their mentality have been unfavourable to the development of surgery, *i.e.*, their general orientation towards the supernatural prevents them from developing a more systematic surgery. Mystical concepts were a vital part of not only medicine but all aspects of life in general, diseases and disorders being attributed to the anger of gods and spirits or the presence of evil demons in the body.

5 - Surgery was not a special field of practice, there was not a definite class of surgeons; the surgeon was the medicine-man, the priest-physician, or just a well-respected elder.

With regard to the first postulate, and even though it might be accurate to say that there is no need for especially extended treatment under primitive conditions, the pathological circumstance to which primitives were exposed to would have been sufficiently numerous to have furnished enough incentive for a more developed surgery.

As to the suggestion that primitives lacked technical expertise, surgery undoubtedly presupposes a considerable manual skill, but many primitive societies, like the Eskimos, show such dexterity and yet are very poor surgeons.

The third postulate is possibly a most accurate one. The great progress in modern surgery was effectively possible by an enormous increase in our knowledge concerning these three fields. However, anaesthetic and aseptic methods are better developed among primitives than usually assumed; on the other hand, as Ackerknecht (1946) points out, the Masai were able to do quite creditable surgery without knowing much about either anaesthesia or asepsis. It is true that anatomical knowledge is an essential condition for successful surgical action, and that such knowledge of primitives is in general very poor.

As to the fourth claim, the direction of the limiting and negative influence which supernaturalistic ideas among primitives exert upon the development of the operator's art is possibly the most satisfactory explanation for the particular character of primitive surgery. This is very clear in the case of the poor anatomical knowledge among primitives, which is not because they lack opportunities to observe anatomical evidence, but primarily because they are not orientated towards such observation. There are tribes in Africa, Asia and Oceania which do perform numerous autopsies in the search for witchcraft principles and yet are just as unaware of the most elementary anatomical conditions as are the non-dissecting tribes. Looking for the supernatural, they just seem not to observe the evident (Ackerknecht, 1967; Sigerist, 1951). The negative influence of supernaturalistic ideas on surgery is also clear in those cases where bodily amputation is dreaded because of its detrimental influence in the future life of the ghost. To this extent, a Central African will not consent to such an operation, as it conflicts with the anticipation of his dismembered spirit. For the same reason, the Polynesian Tanala do not fear death, but are very much afraid of mutilations (Ackerknecht, 1967). In regions where this is a customary form of punishment, people perceptibly dislike undergoing procedures which externally will identify them with criminals, not comprehending that this mutilating or amputating technique might be useful or even life-saving when applied to infected complicated fractures, focuses of septicaemia, tumours, etc. This supernaturalistic orientation also seems to explain why highly complicated operations like trepanation or Caesarean section can coexist with an otherwise undeveloped surgery, a phenomenon impossible in our culture where discoveries are made by logical scientific procedure.

Finally, as the fifth justification emphasizes, we have to bear in mind that an isolated tribal society is a relatively closed community of knowledge and experience, which must be passed on by word of mouth. The limitations of memory restrict the diversity and detail that can be preserved without writing. Moreover, these people did not have a tradition that stressed the importance of the methodical gathering and classification of knowledge in any area.

Nevertheless, as we have seen, all primitive tribes use some kind of wound treatment. The principles are always very similar: herbs or roots, often with astringent or disinfectant qualities, are applied to the wound in form of powders, infusions, or poultices. The results of this treatment are generally described by anthropologists as very good; however, such judgements are based exclusively on the actual healing of the wound, a result which might be explained on the basis of the absence of the virulent strains of bacteria which we have cultivated in our cities and hospitals (Ackerknecht, 1946).

The similarity between methods used in different parts of the world is striking, above all the use of naturally occurring styptic substances to control bleeding, the application of powders and infusions with an astringent or disinfectant action, protective bandaging, heat and massage. The results were often good. On one hand, the methods used were habitually skilful, on the other, primitive man was naturally harder. Finally, highly resistant germs were absent.

Equally universal among primitives is the treatment of fractures. Again, the results of such treatment were generally good and again, judgement on this point is difficult, since well-healed fractures are numerous among wild gibbons and other primates which are not likely to enjoy treatment by professional bonesetters (Ackerknecht, 1967; Sigerist, 1951). Conversely, the considerable skill shown in the application of splints is not always matched by equal care in reduction.

There is no doubt that surgery was born of instinct. A thorn that entered the skin was removed by early man just as it is by animals, as were other foreign bodies as long as they were accessible. An animal licks its wounds and man may well have done it also. He may have stopped a haemorrhage through compression just as he must have practised bleeding at an early stage: scratching became scarification and sucking became cupping.

As to the practise of incision, it is not as widespread as the above mentioned, but it is still fairly frequent, particularly the opening of boils and abscesses.

The amputation of limbs severely torn by wild beasts or crushed by falling trees or rocks undoubtedly was undertaken by prehistoric man as a desperate measure. In this case, as in many others, surgery was an action of last resort. Interpreting archaeological examples of amputation is quite difficult, especially because there are not enough cases from any one geographical area for statistical analysis of patterning in terms of affected limbs, gender, age at death, etc. Among modern primitive tribes, the main reasons for amputation are either judicial-related, *i.e.*, punishment after some offence (as seen in Polynesia or amid the Seneca Indians), or ritual-related, essentially the mourning of a death (as seen in New Guinea and Melanesia). The archaeological record of amputation is scant, but such records of trepanation are abundant. When the surgical risks of trepanation and amputation are compared, it is surprising that, on the evidence available, the former appears to have been a more common surgical manoeuvre than the latter; nevertheless, this may be explained on the basis of the relative ease of recognition of trepanation and the likely difficulty of acknowledgment of amputation.

Trepanation is a feature of primitive surgery widely spread in space and time. That prehistoric humans, using the most rudimentary instruments, were able to bore open a human skull allowing the patient to survive, is an incredible medical achievement. Simultaneously, the existence of such a complicated operation among tribes who otherwise limit their surgery to wound treatment, bone-setting and bloodletting, constitutes a striking contradiction. The survival rate observed, plus the discovery of skulls sometimes trepanned more than once, are very good proofs of the skill of the early surgeons and also of the common practise of this operation in prehistoric times. Nevertheless, if the success of this operation is explainable where it is a routine procedure, its genesis and independent development are hard to understand.

It is imperative to consider the conditions under which this operation would have been performed. Even though far from aseptic, they were in all probability free from many hazards of contamination and infection.

Furthermore, we cannot ignore the abundant evidence of technical skill on the part of the operator. Indeed, it is not surprising that manual skill and precise manipulation was applied to surgery in cultures where ceramics, textile weaving, stone working and metallurgy were later developed.

Nonetheless, why such ability was mainly restricted to this operation is difficult to explain. Maybe we should focus on the fact that prehistoric humans lived in a considerably dangerous and hazardous environment where accidents, hunting and battles would have resulted in frequent head trauma. There must have been a considerable amount of experience based knowledge about weapons, blows and wounds. A blow to the head could have easily revealed the bare skull, and if left untreated, exposed bone dries out and dies. The demarcation between living and dead bone is quite clear – sections appear pale and bloodless if kept clean and covered, but black and necrotic if the blood pigments oxidize with air. It is therefore relatively simple to take a sharp flint and scrape away at the dead bone, thus speeding the closure of the wound.

I think this leads us to the conclusion that trepanation could have been invented out of daily experience. Even though the evidence for magico-religious implications appears in some occasions convincing (science and magic were indistinguishable in its early stages, and being so it is difficult to differentiate between ritual and medical motives), it is equally clear that the operation was also a therapeutic procedure done to correct a serious medical problem. Reasons for trepanning certainly varied from place to place and time to time. Even in present day primitive cultures the reasons offered are not always the same: the Kisii motive, for instance, is to relieve headache after a blow; yet a few hundred miles away, the Lugbara motive is to let out an evil spirit.

As to caesarean section, while its antiquity is definitely established under early Roman civilisation, it is however impossible to ascertain when it was first performed, given that for obvious reasons it is impossible to obtain an archaeological record of such a procedure.

Anthropologists and Archaeologists do not agree upon the origins of circumcision. Some believe that it is a feature of a heliolithic culture which spread over much of the world over 15,000 years ago, while others claim that it originated independently within different regions and cultures. We now know that many of the natives Columbus found in the New World were circumcised, the operation also being practised in the Near East, among several African tribes, the Moslem peoples of India and South East Asia, and Australian Aborigines. While some African people perform it at birth, Moslems perform it in early adult life as a rite of passage, puberty or marriage, and in Judaic societies the ritual takes place on the eighth day after birth, being viewed as an outward sign of a covenant between God and man. In Ancient Egypt captured warriors were often circumcised before being condemned to slavery. Scholars have suggested that this procedure could represent a mark of cultural identity, akin to a tattoo or a body piercing, or alternatively a fertility rite, which would seem reasonable as the penis was believed to be inhabited by powers that produced life. Evidence of a connection with harvests is also found in Nicaragua, where blood from the operation was mixed with maize and eaten during the ceremony. The true origins of circumcision will never be found, but we can possibly claim that all the theories described here are likely to be partly right.

It is almost unconceivable that our prehistoric ancestors did not use extraction of teeth as an effective method of treating toothache, but it is difficult to prove it by examining skeletons, in view of the fact that extraction does not leave evidence distinguishable from natural loss of teeth.

There are numerous tribes which never open an abscess, but do amputate and mutilate fingers, toes and genitalia quite extensively if their religious rites or ideas concerning punishment indicate such procedures. These operations could hardly develop under such circumstances which produced negative associations with surgery. Some of these ethnographic examples probably represent the unusual cases seen by scientists, writers and travellers over wide areas and during many years of residence. It is not fair to claim them all as regular practices, or to suppose that any one man knows all of them, although many of them are definitely of everyday use. On the other hand we must bear in mind that the native knows much more than we have been able to find out; primitives are careful to guard the knowledge inherited from their fathers or tutors, and as Harley (1970) states, in some cases they absolutely refuse to divulge the secret of a remedy successfully used in a particularly difficult case.

As to the cutting for bladder stone, the simplest procedure would have been to cut down on to the base of the bladder through the perineum, involving the use of no special instruments, merely a knife and a hook to help extract the stone. This technique was most possibly the one practised by our primitive ancestors. Regrettably, there is not much more we can state about this procedure in prehistoric times, its *modus operandi* remaining a matter of conjecture.

Prehistoric surgery demonstrates progress in surgical proficiency to an impressive level of technical ability considering Stone Age instrumentation. Equally, the doctrinal and theoretical base for ancient practices was conceivably fantastic, essentially supernatural and unquestionably pre-scientific. Still, a blend of technical skill, some degree of empirical knowledge, and traditional authority produced a successful healing in many cases of injury and illness.

In my opinion, the surgical achievements of prehistoric and primitive humans are unquestionably impressive in view of their lack of anatomical knowledge and basic instrumentation. A combination of the primitive surgeon's technical skills and empirical information must have brought about successful restoration of health in many cases of trauma and illness. Primitive surgery was a last resort rather than an elective procedure;

nevertheless, today's surgical techniques have their roots in ancient knowledge and are part of the continuing saga of medical evolution.

III APPENDIX
Surgical History of Ancient Civilisations

At the most remote period of recorded history, the character of surgery was obviously mainly magico-religious. Nevertheless, much of it was rational, and there was much accumulated knowledge about different diseases and how to treat them. Here is a very brief synopsis of the surgical history of ancient civilisations.

- ANCIENT EGYPT

A great deal is known about the surgery of Ancient Egyptians thanks not only to objects which have been excavated from tombs and temples but also to the large number of documents that have survived, showing us that medicine was already becoming a science as well as an art. In fact, the Egyptians enjoyed great fame as physicians, and these specialists occupied positions of great honour and renown (Bishop, 1960). Egyptian medicine doctrine reflected their dualistic culture – one facet was practical and naturalistic, the other mystical and folkloristic, the two approaches to healing often being confused. The practice of mummification might have been an indirect contribution to surgery in the sense that it gave physicians the opportunity to learn anatomy.

A number of medical documents have come to us in the form of papyrus rolls. The main ones range from about 2,000 to 1,200 BC, but the knowledge and ideas they contain must relate to a considerably older period, probably five or six thousand years ago. From a surgical point of view, the most interesting is the Edwin Smith Papyrus, a roll of about five metres in length containing descriptions of forty-eight cases of injuries, wounds, fractures, dislocations and tumours that establishes the oldest surgical work known to mankind. The advices given are entirely rational and magic-free, being organised from symptoms to examination, diagnosis, prognosis and finally treatment. This papyrus clearly shows that the Egyptians had some anatomical knowledge and considerable experience of war surgery.

- ANCIENT BABYLON AND ASSYRIA

In Ancient Babylon and Assyria, medicine had also reached a high stage of development. In the second millennium BC, one of the earliest kings of Babylon, Hammurabi, assembled a comprehensive code of laws related to medical practice which shows us that medicine and surgery were exceedingly structured professions, fees being regulated and penalties laid down for failure.

The library of Ashurbanipal, king of Assyria in the seventh century, consists of thirty thousand tablets of baked clay bearing cuneiform writing, eight hundred of which are medical texts.

- ANCIENT INDIA

The medical history of India contains much legendary lore and it is strangely inconsistent, but it is particularly interesting. It involved witchcraft and demonology, alongside an inaccurate anatomical knowledge, a high level of skill was still indisputably achieved. Actually, some operations described in Indian texts (such as the cure for anal fistula), did not come into use in the rest of the world until the late Medieval period. Other surgical operations thought to have been practised by the Ancient Indians consisted of tonsillectomy, removal of bladder stone, operations on tumours of the neck, rhinoplasty and caesarean section. Blood vessels were sewn, fractures reduced, limbs amputated and iron prostheses provided.

- ANCIENT CHINA

The alleged father of Chinese medicine was the Emperor Shen Nung, who lived about 5,000 years ago and who discovered a large number of remedies and poisons. Similarly to other early civilisations, Chinese medicine gradually escaped from the control of magic and superstition. The cause of all diseases was thought to be some disturbance of the two principles of Yin (feminine) and Yang (masculine), and the principal means adopted to restore such balance was counter-irritation by acupuncture – introduction of long, fine needles into the body at various specified points, in order to remove obstructions and allowing the bad secretions to escape.

By around 2,500 BC surgeons made incisions through the skin, tied blood vessels, sutured tendons, exposed the brain and spinal cord, cleansed the stomach and intestines. A particularly popular procedure was castration, performed in order to produce eunuchs for the Imperial court.

IV <u>TABLE OF FIGURES</u>

Figure 10 – Both these femora from central Murray (Australia) have sites of infection around their amputated stumps. These may have resulted from the operation itself or were the reason for the amputation (Webb, 1995)

Figure 11 – Central Australian Aborigine with an amputated right leg who was taken to use a crutch (Webb, 1995)

Figure 12 – Methods of trepanning: (1) scraping; (2) grooving; (3) boring and cutting; (4) intersecting incisions (Lisowski, 1967)

Figure 13 – Peruvian skull showing three trepanations (Mann, 1991)

Figure 14 – Peruvian skull showing healed trepanation – the opening shows smooth borders and a closed diplöe (Chege et al., 1996)

Figure 15 – Healed trepanation almost in the centre of the frontal bone of a Neolithic Danish skull (Bennike, 1985)

Figure 16 – Partially healed trepanation on the coronal suture between the left parietal bone and the frontal bone of an Iron Age Danish skull (Bennike, 1985)

Figure 17 – Neolithic skull from the Pyrenees displaying perforations caused by a multiple myeloma (Brothwell, 1981)

Figure 18 – Trepanation by cutting on a child from Peru. There is clear evidence of association with trauma - long circular fracture and radiating fracture extending from the former. There is no evidence of healing (Ortner and Putschar, 1981)

Figure 19 – Photographs from a video showing a trepanation of an African child after injury to the frontal region: (a) the patient prior to trepanation; (b) the patient with the skull exposed during trepanation; (c) the patient post-trepanation with bandages (Rawlings and Rossitch, 1994)

Figure 20 – Superior view of the cranium exhibiting oval trepanation (Mogle and Zias, 1995)

Figure 21 – Two Kenyan skulls trepanned in life with two knives, two scrapers with curved tips, and one saw. The skull on the left has been holed by scraping, the one on the right by sawing (Margetts, 1967)

Figure 22 – "Hat On" (Margetts, 1967)

Figure 23 – "Hat Off" (Margetts, 1967)

Figure 24 – Antero-posterior skull x-ray of the patient (Margetts, 1967)

Figure 25 – Lateral skull x-ray of the patient (Margetts, 1967)

Figure 26– Sincipital T scar (Young, 1944)

Figure 27 – Atrophy of the skull in the region of sagittal and lambdoid sutures (Ortner and Putschar, 1981)

Figure 28 – Medicine-man from Zimbabwe reading the divine bones for diagnosis of the cause of illness (Sigerist, 1951)

Figure 29 – Central Australian medicine-man (Spencer and Gillen, 1899)

Figure 30 – Navajo medicine-man (Sigerist, 1951)

Figure 31 – Siberian medicine-man (Sigerist, 1951)

Figure 32 – Nigerian medicine-man (Sigerist, 1951)

Figure 33 – Trepan instruments from Kenya (Margetts, 1967)

Figure 34 – Copper needle, silver needle and copper pin with loop head from Naqada, Egypt (4500-3000 BC). Below is an unprovenanced bone needle case containing fifteen copper alloy needles from Egypt (1550-1069) (Nunn, 1996)

V <u>BIBLIOGRAPHY</u>

1. ACKERKNECHT, E. H. [ed.] (1967) – "Primitive Surgery", **Diseases in Antiquity**, Illinois: Charles C. Thomas.

2. ____ (1982) – **A Short History of Medicine**, Baltimore: John Hopkins University Press.

3. ALT, K. *et al.* (1997) – "Evidence for Stone Age Cranial Surgery", **Nature**, 387: 360.

4. ASHLEY-MONTAGU, M. (1937) – "The Origin of Subincision in Australia", **Oceania**, 8: 193-207.

5. ARNOTT, R., FINGER, S. and SMITH, C. (2003) – **Trepanation: History – Discovery – Theory**, Lisse: Swets & Zeitlinger.

6. BANDELIER, A. (1904) – "Aboriginal Trephining in Bolivia", **American Anthropologist**, 6: 440-447.

7. BARBER, C. (1929) – "Immediate and Eventual Features of Healing in Amputated Bones", **Annals of Surgery**, 90: 985-992.

8. BARBER, C. and CLEVELAND, O. (1934) – "Ultimate Anatomical Modifications in Amputation Stumps", **Journal of Bone and Joint Surgery**, 16: 394-400.

9. BENNIKE, P. (1985) – **Palaeopathology of Danish Skeletons: a Comparative Study of Demography, Disease and Injury**, Copenhagen: Akademisk Forlag.

10. BENNIKE, P. and FREDEBO, L. (1986) – "Dental treatment in the Stone Age", **Bulletin of the History of Dentistry**, 34 (2): 81-87.

11. BENNION, E. (1979) – **Antique Medical Instruments**, London: Sotheby's Publications.

12. BISHOP, W. (1959) – **A History of Surgical Dressing**, Chesterfield, Robinson & Sons.

13. ____ (1960) – **The Early History of Surgery**, New York: Barnes and Noble.

14. BLOOM, A. (1995) – "Amputation of the Hand in the 3,600 year old Skeletal Remains of an Adult Male: the 1st Case reported from Israel", **International Journal of Osteoarchaeolgy**, 5: 188-191.

15. BROWN, G. (1910) – **Melanesians and Polynesians**, London: Macmillan.

16. BYNUN, W. and PORTER, R. [eds.] (1993) – **Companion Encyclopaedia of the History of Medicine**, vol.1, London: Routeledge.

17. BROTHWELL, D. (1981) – **Digging up Bones**, New York: Cornell University Press.

18. BROTHWELL, D. and SANDISON, A. (1967) – **Diseases in Antiquity**, Illinois: C. Thomas.

19. CALDER, R. (1958) – **Medicine and Man – The Story of the Art and Science of Healing**, London: George Allen & Unwin.

20. CAPASSO, L. and TOTA, G. (1996) – "Possible Therapy for Headaches in Ancient Times", **International Journal of Osteoarchaeology**, 6: 316-319.

21. CASTIGLIONI, A. (1947) – **A History of Medicine**, New York: Alfred A. Knopf.

22. CHEGE, N. *et al.* (1996) – "Imaging Evaluation of Skull Trepanation using Radiography and CT", **International Journal of Osteoarchaeology**, 6: 249-258.

23. CRUMP, J. (1901) – "Trephining in the South Seas", **Journal of the Royal Anthropological Institution**, 31:167.

24. DeBAKEY, M. (1991) – "A Surgical Perspective", **Annals of Surgery**, 213: 499-531.

25. DERUMS, V. (1979) – "Extensive Trepanation of the Skull in Ancient Latvia", **Bulletin of the History of Medicine**, 53: 459-464.

26. DRIBERG, J. (1923) – **The Lango**, London: Fisher Unwin.

27. DUNSMUIR, W. and GORDON, E. (1999) – "The History of Circumcision", **British Journal of Urology**, 83: 1-12.

28. ELLIS, E. (1946) – **Ancient Anodynes. Primitive Anaesthesia and Allied Conditions**, London: Heinemann.

29. ELLIS, H. (2001) – **A History of Surgery**, London: Greenwich Medical Media.

30. FILER, J. (1995) – **Egyptian Bookshelf – Disease**, London: British Museum Press.

31. FORTUINE, R. (1985) – "Lancets of Stone: Traditional Methods of Surgery among the Alaska Natives", **Arctic Anthropology**, 22: 23-45.

32. GAIRDNER, D. (1949) – "The Fate of the Foreskin. A Study of Circumcision", **British Medical Journal**, 2: 1433-1437.

33. GARRISON, F. (1929) – **An Introduction to the History of Medicine**, London: W. B. Saunders.

34. GOLDSMITH, W. (1945) – "Trepanation and the Catlin Mark", **American Antiquity**, 10: 348-352.

35. GUTHRIE, D. (1958) – **A History of Medicine**, London: Thomas Nelson.

36. HAEGER, Knut (1988) – **The Illustrated History of Surgery**, London: Harold Starke.

37. HARLEY, G. (1970) – **Native African Medicine**, London: Frank Cass.

38. HART, G. (1983) – **Disease in Ancient Man**, Ontario: Clarke Irwin.

39. HILTON-SIMPSON, (1913) – "Some Arab and Shawia Remedies and Notes on the Trepanning of the Skull in Algeria", **Journal of the Royal Anthropological Institution**, 43: 715.

40. HORSLEY, V. (1888) – "Trephining in the Neolithic Period", **Journal of the Royal Anthropological Institution**, 17:100.

41. HULTKRANTZ, Ã. (2003) – "The Relation Between Medical States and Soul Beliefs Among Tribal People", **Medicine Across Cultures: History and Practice of Medicine in Non-Western Cultures**, London: Kluwer Academic Publishers, 385-395.

42. JANSEN, J and GREEN, E. (2003) – "Continuity, Change and Challenge in African Medicine", **Medicine Across Cultures: History and Practice of Medicine in Non-Western Cultures**, London: Kluwer Academic Publishers, 1-27.

43. JONES, A. (1977) – "Medical Practise and Tribal Communities", **Health and Disease in Tribal Societies**, Oxford: Elsevier, 243-268.

44. KARSTEN, R. (1926) – **The Civilisation of the South American Indians**, London: Dawson.

45. KERRIDGE, I. and LOWE, M. (1995) – "Bloodletting: the Story of a Therapeutic Technique", **Medical Journal of Australia**, 163: 631-633.

46. KIRKUP, J. (1981) – "The History and Evolution of Surgical Instruments I - Introduction" **Annals of the Royal College of Surgeons of England**, 63: 280-285.

47. ____ (1982) – "The History and Evolution of Surgical Instruments II – Origins: Function, Carriage, Manufacture", **Annals of the Royal College of Surgeons of England**, 64: 125-130.

48. ____ (1985) – "The History and Evolution of Surgical Instruments IV: Probes and their Allies", **Annals of the Royal College of Surgeons of England**, 67: 56-60.

49. ____ (1986) – "The History and Evolution of Surgical Instruments V: Needles and their Penetrating Derivatives", **Annals of the Royal College of Surgeons of England**, 68: 29-33.

50. ____ (1993) – "From Flint to Stainless Steel: Observations on Surgical Instrument Composition", **Annals of the Royal College of Surgeons of England**, 75: 365-374.

51. ____ (1995) – "The History and Evolution of Surgical Instruments VI: The Surgical Blade, from Fingernail to Ultrasound", **Annals of the Royal College of Surgeons of England**, 77: 380-388.

52. ____ (1996) - "The History and Evolution of Surgical Instruments VII: Spring Forceps (Tweezers), Hooks and Simple Retractors", **Annals of the Royal College of Surgeons of England**, 78: 514-525.

53. KIRKUP, J. and LEWIS, G. (1977) – "Beliefs and Behaviour in Disease", **Health and Disease in Tribal Societies**, Oxford: Elsevier, 227-242.

54. KOTTEK, S. (2003) – "Medicine in Ancient Hebrew and Jewish Cultures", **Medicine Across Cultures: History and Practice of Medicine in Non-Western Cultures**, London: Kluwer Academic Publishers, 305-324.

55. LILLIE, M. (1998) – "Cranial Surgery dates back to Mesolithic", **Nature**, 391: 854.

56. LISOWSKI, F. (1967) – "Prehistoric and Early Historic Trepanations", **Diseases in Antiquity**, Illinois: C. Thomas, 651-672.

57. LUCIER, C. (1971) – "Medical Practises and Human Anatomical Knowledge among the Noatak Eskimos", **Ethnology**, 10: 251-260.

58. MACONI, G. (1991) – **Storia della Medicina e della Chirurgia**, Milano: Casa Editrice Ambrosiana.

59. MACPHERSON, C. and MACPHERSON, L. (2003) – "When Healing Cultures Collide: A Case from the Pacific", **Medicine Across Cultures: History and Practice of Medicine in Non-Western Cultures**, London: Kluwer Academic Publishers, 191-207.

60. MAGNER, L. (1992) – "The Art and Science of Surgery", **A History of Medicine**, New York: Marcel Dekker, 279-304.

61. MAJNO, G. (1975) – **The Healing Hand. Man and Wound in the Ancient World**, Cambridge: Harvard University Press.

62. MALLEGNI, F. and VALASSINA, A. (1996) – "Secondary Bone Changes to a Cranium Trepanation in a Neolithic Man discovered at Trasano, South Italy", **International Journal of Osteoarchaelogy**, 6: 506-511.

63. MALLIN, R. (1976) – "A Trephined Skull from Iran", **Bulletin of the New York Academy of Medicine**, 52(7): 782-787.

64. MANN, G. (1991) – "Chronic Ear Disease as a Possible Reason for Trepanation", **International Journal of Osteoarchaeology**, 1: 165-168.

65. MARGETTS, E. (1967) – "Trepanation of the Skull by the Medicine-man of Primitive Cultures with Particular Reference to Present Day Native East African Practise", **Diseases in Antiquity**, Illinois: C. Thomas, 673-695.

66. MAYS, S. (1996) – "Healed limb Amputations in Human Osteoarchaeology and their Causes: a Case Study from Ipswich, UK", **International Journal of Osteoarchaeology**, 6: 101-113.

67. MCGREW, R. (1985) – **Encyclopaedia of Medical History**, London: Macmillan Press.

68. MEHL-MADRONA, L. (2003) – "Native American Medicine: Herbal Pharmacology, Therapies, and Elder Care", **Medicine Across Cultures: History and Practice of Medicine in Non-Western Cultures**, London: Kluwer Academic Publishers, 209-224.

69. MENDOZA, R. (2003) – "Lords of the Medicine Bag: Medical Science and Traditional Practice in Ancient Peru and South America", **Medicine Across**

Cultures: History and Practice of Medicine in Non-Western Cultures, London: Kluwer Academic Publishers, 225-257.

70. MOGLE, P. and ZIAS, J. (1995) – "Trepanation as a Possible Treatment for Scurvy in a Middle Bronze Age Skeleton", **International Journal of Osteoarchaeology**, 5: 77-81.

71. NUNN, J. (1996) – **Ancient Egyptian Medicine**, London: British Museum Press.

72. OAKLEY, K. P., BROOKE, W. M. A., AKESTER, A. R., and BROTHWELL, D. R. (1959) – "Contributions on trepanning or Trepanation in Ancient and Modern Times", **Man**, 59: 93-106.

73. ORTNER, D. and PUTSCHAR, W. (1981) – **Identification of Pathological Conditions in Human Skeletal Remains**, Washington: Smithsonian Institute Press.

74. ORTNER, D. and THEOBALD, G. (1993) – "Diseases in the Pre-Roman World", **The Cambridge History of Human Disease**, Cambridge: CUP, 247-261.

75. PARKER, S.; ROBERTS, C. and MANCHESTER, K. (1986) – "A Review of British Trepanations with Reports on Two New Cases", **OSSA**, 12: 141-158.

76. PARRY, W. (1917) – "The Art of Trephining among Prehistoric and Primitive people", **Journal of the British Archaeological Association**, 22: 33-68.

77. PERSSON, O. (1977) – "A Trepanned Skull from the Gillhög passage-grave at Barsebäck in West Scania (Southern Sweden)", **OSSA**, ¾: 53-61.

78. PIGGOTT, S. (1940) – "A Trepanned Skull of the Beaker Period from Dorset and the Practise of Trepanning in Prehistoric Europe", **Proceedings of the Prehistoric Society**, 6: 112-132.

79. POLUNIN, I. (1977) – "Some Characteristics of Tribal People", **Health and Disease in Tribal Societies**, Oxford: Elsevier, 5-24.

80. PRIORESCHI, P. (1991) – "Possible Reasons for Neolithic Skull Trephining", **Perspectives in Biology and Medicine**, 34(2): 296-303.

81. ____ (1995) – **A History of Medicine: Primitive and Ancient Medicine**, Omaha: Horatius Press.

82. RAWLINGS, C. and ROSSITCH, E. (1994) – "The History of Trephination in Africa with a Discussion of its Current Status and Continuing Practice", **Surgical Neurology**, 41: 507-513.

83. RHODES, P. (1985) – **An Outline History of Medicine**, London: Butterworths.

84. RICHARDS, G. (1995) – "Earliest Cranial Surgery in North America", **American Journal of Physical Anthropology**, 98: 203-209.

85. ROBERTS, C. and MANCHESTER, K. (1997) – **The Archaeology of Disease**, Gloucestershire: Sutton Publishing Limited.

86. ROGERS, S. (1985) – **Primitive Surgery: Skills before Science**, Springfield: Charles C. Thomas.

87. RUTKOW, I. (1993) – **Surgery: An Illustrated History**, London: Norman Publishing.

88. ____ (1998) – **American Surgery: An Illustrated History**, New York: Lippincott-Raven.

89. SACHS, E. (1952) – **The History and Development of Neurosurgical History**, London: Cassell and Co.

90. SHAFIK, A. and ELSEESY, W. (2003) – "Medicine in Ancient Egypt", **Medicine Across Cultures: History and Practice of Medicine in Non-Western Cultures**, London: Kluwer Academic Publishers, 27-47.

91. SIGERIST, H. (1951) – **A History of Medicine. Volume I: Primitive and Archaic Medicine**, New York: Oxford University Press.

92. SPENCER, B. and GILLEN, F. (1899) – **The Native Tribes of Central Australia**, London: MacMillan and Co.

93. STEVENS, G. and WAKLEY, J. (1993) – "Diagnosis Criteria for Identification of Sea-Shell as a Trepanation Implement", **International Journal of Osteoarchaeology**, 3: 167-176.

94. STEWART, T. (1958) – "Stone Age Skull Surgery", **Smithsonian Institution Annual Report**, Washington: Smithsonian Institute Press.

95. STONE, J. and MILES, M. (1990) – "Skull Trepanation among the Early Indians of Canada and the United States", **Neurosurgery**, 26: 1015-1020.

96. TURK, J. (1983) – "Bleeding and Cupping", **Annals of the Royal College of Surgeons of England**, 65(2): 128-131.

97. VARA-LOPÉZ, D. (1949) – **La Craniectomía através de los Siglos**, Valladolid: Sever-Cuesta.

98. VIESCA, C. (2003) – "Medicine in Ancient Mesoamerica", **Medicine Across Cultures: History and Practice of Medicine in Non-Western Cultures**, London: Kluwer Academic Publishers, 259-283.

99. VOGEL, V. (1970) – **American Indian Medicine**, Norman: University of Oklahoma Press.

100. WANGESTEEN, O. (1967) – "Some Highlights in the History of Amputation", **Bulletin of the History of Medicine**, 41(2): 97-131.

101. WANGENSTEEN, O. and WANGENSTEEN, S. (1978) – **The Rise of Surgery. From Empiric Craft to Scientific Discipline**, Minneapolis: University of Minnesota Press.

102. WEBB, S. (1988) – "Two Possible Cases of Trepanation from Australia", **American Journal of Physical Anthropology**, 75: 541-548.

103. ____ (1995) – **Palaeopathology of Aboriginal Australians**, Cambridge: Cambridge University Press.

104. WEBB, T. (1933) – "Aboriginal Medical Practise in East Arnhem Land", **Oceania**, 4: 91-98.

105. WELLS, C. (1964) – **Bones, Bodies and Disease**, London: Thames and Hudson.
106. WESTON-DAVIES, W. (1989) – "The Surgical Instrument Maker: A Historical Perspective", **Journal of the Royal Society of Medicine**, 82: 40-60.

107. WYATT, J. (1994) – "The Roots of North American Medicine", **Indian Life Magazine**, 15:3.

108.   YOUNG, J. (1944) – **Caesarean Section: The History and Development of the Operation from Earliest Times**, London: H. K. Lewis.

109.   ZIAS, J. and NUMEROFF, K. (1987) – "Operative Dentistry in the 2nd Century BC", **Journal of the American Dental Association**, 114: 665-666.

110.   ZIAS, J. and POMERANZ, S. (1992) – "Serial Craniectomies for Intracranial Infection 5.5 Millennia Ago", **International Journal of Osteoarchaeology**, 2: 183-186.

111.   ZYVANOVIC, S. (1982) – **Ancient Diseases. The Elements of Palaeopathology**, London: Methuen & Co.

www.ingramcontent.com/pod-product-compliance
Lightning Source LLC
Chambersburg PA
CBHW061301270326
41932CB00029B/3425